BLESSED ARE THE
CAREGIVERS

A Daily Book of Comfort and Cheer

by

Bethany Knight

D0401445

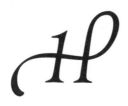

Hartman Publishing

Credits

Managing Editor: Susan Alvare
Developmental Editor: Kristin Dyche
Interior Design: Thad Castillo/Susan Alvare
Cover Design: Thad Castillo
Cover Illustration: Steven Verriest
Page Layout: Susan Alvare
Proofreader: Joey Tulino

Copyright © 2001 by Bethany Knight. All rights reserved. No part of this book may be used or reproduced in any manner whatsoever without written permission from the publisher.

All bibliographic information and credit lines not listed on the pages on which the information first appears are listed in the References section, which begins on page 442.

Excerpt from "A Father's Story" from *The Times Are Never So Bad* by Andre Dubus. Reprinted by permission of David R. Godine, Publisher, Inc. Copyright © 1983 by Andre Dubus.

ISBN 1-888343-53-2

For information contact:

HARTMAN **H** PUBLISHING INC.

Hartman Publishing, Inc.
8529-A Indian School NE
Albuquerque, NM 87112
1-800-999-9534

hartmanonline.com

BLESSED ARE THE

CAREGIVERS

A Daily Book of Comfort and Cheer

by

Bethany Knight

Foreword

I first met Bethany Knight at an airport. She was to be the keynote speaker at the Portman conference, a day-long celebration of CNAs and the work they do with persons suffering dementia. I had volunteered to chauffeur, hoping to learn something in the precious moments that I would have her to myself.

I had second thoughts about whether or not I should have volunteered to pick someone up in my dearly-loved-but-definitely-used old car, "Mary Jo." What would this nationally-known speaker think of an organization that sent such a courier?

Traffic was unusually heavy that day. I had not left work as early as I had planned. The short-term parking was full. Without enough time left to seek out a shuttle, I parked in the long-term area and started walking. As I walked, I became more excited, but also more anxious. What would I say to this person? Would she see me (a ridiculous thought, as I carried a 2'x3' bright orange sign)? Should I have her wait by the doors while I get the car?

I checked the monitor at the ticket counter and headed for the gate. Her flight was arriving on time. I had been told I could meet her at the baggage claim, but somehow that offended my sense of hospitality. No, I must meet her at the gate with my bright orange sign. Still plenty of time.

I got to the gate only to find a change had been made. She would now be arriving at the opposite end of the terminal, still on time. I once again started walking and came to a gate that didn't look like one. There were no planes, no check-in counter, and outside was a street with taxis and shuttles. I stood, for what seemed like forever, as several shuttles unloaded. Passengers glanced at my sign, some even smiled, but they kept on walking. More shuttles unloaded, all without producing Bethany. Everyone was gone, even the skycaps.

By now I had several doubts. Did I misread the monitors? Did I have the right airline? Was I even at the right airport?

Who was I to think that I should be the one to pick her up in the first place?

As I walked into a nearby restroom, I heard another van pull up. I stepped out of that restroom, my sign tucked under my arm, almost the instant that Bethany walked in at the gate. She couldn't have read the sign at that angle, but she must have sensed this lost-looking soul was looking for her. Our eyes met, we hugged, and Bethany said, "Tell me about yourself."

A friendship was born at that airport, one that I believe God had designed a very long time ago. When I met Bethany, I felt as if we had been friends most of my life. I knew in a moment: here was someone who completely understood my passion in life, caring for "old souls." She shared this passion, and acknowledged the vision I have for a better, holistic, person-centered approach to eldercare in America.

Those moments of having Bethany to yourself are here. She will speak to you as she has to me—because she is real, because of her unshadowed vision for a better world for caregivers and those we care for, because she believes, as I do, that our work is holy, ordained by God.

Her words will meet you in the moments of pain, doubt, fear, celebration, anticipation, spontaneity, and purely unaltered joy that all caregivers experience, whether a CNA, a nurse, a housekeeper, a food service worker, or even an activities director like me.

My journey with Bethany has been personal, growing, spiritual, and most of all, blessed. I know that yours will be, too. Treasure the journey.

Jill R. Trewin, April, 2001

Jill Trewin is currently the Resident Services Manager at Father Murray Nursing Center in Center Line, Michigan.

Dedication

Standing at the foot of his modest grave, I placed a garland of gardenias across the stone inscribed "Bede Griffiths." A Roman Catholic monk, Bede lived as an Indian in India for 35 years, a witness of the unity and harmony he wished to forge between East and West—between all peoples. He lived and was buried at Shantivanam (Peace Forest), the ashram he founded in southern India.

> We have to discover the inner relationship between...different aspects of Truth and unite them in ourselves. I have to be a Hindu, a Buddhist, a Jain, a Parsee, a Sikh, a Muslim, and a Jew, as well as a Christian, if I am to know the Truth and to find the point of reconciliation in all religion...the goal of each religion is the same.

Sitting in the sweet heat of a December day in northern India one week later, I listened to His Holiness the Dalai Lama, the Buddhist exiled Tibetan leader, talk about how he found the Beatitudes of the Bible so beautiful. He compared them to the teachings of his own religious tradition.

> We must love without attachment, (blessed are the poor) with compassion and kindness, (blessed are those who show mercy) this is very important. Attachment based on one's mental projection makes one blind. Too much attachment leads to hate, but too much expectation without attachment makes feelings towards enemies and friends equal, (blessed are the peacemakers).

On a plane that same year, a young wood carver shared his Bahá'í faith and teachings from Abdu'l Baha, and gave me a book.

> Religion should unite all hearts and cause wars and disputes to vanish from the face of the earth; it should give birth to spirituality, and bring light and life to every soul. If religion becomes a cause of dislike, hatred and division it would be better to be without it, and to withdraw from such a religion would be truly a religious act. For it is clear that the purpose of a remedy is to cure, but if the remedy only aggravates the complaint, it had better

be left alone. Any religion which is not a cause of love and unity is no religion.

Last summer in Jackson, Mississippi, Hazel Williams, a certified nursing assistant with the heart and voice of a giant, opened a meeting with other CNAs by singing a rousing spiritual. We clung to her rich, swelling voice as it carried us across time and space. An aide 26 of her 45 years, Hazel could tame a mountain lion with her love alone. The Mississippi aides continue to meet monthly by telephone, with "Hazel Leads Prayer" a fixed agenda item. Everyone knows Hazel's prayers are heard.

Bede Griffiths.
His Holiness the Dalai Lama.
Abdu'l Baha.
Hazel Williams.

Traveling these dazzling moments like rocks across the river, I have heard one single message: of a loving, whole, peaceful and just world. And nowhere does this message ring more brilliantly than in the lives of America's caregivers.

Caregivers are great lovers of life, with faith like a furnace. Regardless of the tenets, their faith burns within and fuels words and deeds over long lifetimes of giving beyond measure.

Employers are forever seeking the secrets for recruiting these extraordinary souls. I suggest the formula lies in recognition of their faith life. What makes someone care for a stranger with the tenderness reserved for a family member? Faith. Faith in a loving, whole, peaceful and just world.

It is in this spirit of recognition for the saints among us, and with great affection, I dedicate this book. Based on the Beatitudes, may this little book feed many a furnace!

Introduction
Gift of Good Things That Are Useful

What are the Beatitudes?

Derived from the Latin beatus meaning blessed or happy, the Beatitudes are the lines that begin Jesus' famous Sermon on the Mount, found in the fifth chapter, verses three through twelve, of the Gospel according to Matthew.

But what are the Beatitudes? Eight or nine teachings that name the virtues leading to a blessed life. The Beatitudes are a recipe for right living, for a way of life that includes good works and blessed feelings. Sounds like caregiving to me.

Within the Russian Orthodox Church, the term Beatitudes has been translated as "Gift of Good Things That Are Useful." A two part sentence, the first clause states the cause for blessing, the second half is the benediction, the promise or reward.

The Beatitudes

> January: Blessed are the poor in spirit, for theirs is the kingdom of heaven.
> February: Blessed are those who mourn, for they shall be comforted.
> March: Blessed are the gentle, for they shall inherit the earth.
> April: Blessed are they who hunger and thirst for holiness, for they shall be satisfied.
> May: Blessed are the merciful, for they shall receive mercy.
> June: Blessed are the pure in heart, for they shall see God.
> July: Blessed are the peacemakers, for they shall be called children of God.
> August: Blessed are those who have been persecuted for the sake of righteousness, for theirs is the kingdom of heaven.

Because we have 12 months, I have extended the Beatitudes by including verses thirteen to sixteen of the Sermon:

September: Rejoice and be glad, for your reward in heaven is great.

October: You are the salt of the earth.

November: You are the light of the world.

December: Let your light so shine that they may know you by your good works.

Ester Mary Walker wrote the *Beatitudes for the Aged*, a poignant poem saluting caregivers, but lacking the second half of the Beatitude classic form, the benediction. Perhaps this book will provide Ester's missing benedictions.

Beatitudes for the Aged

Blessed are they
Who understand
My faltering step
And palsied hand.
Blessed are they
Who know today
My ears must strain
To catch what they say.
Blessed are they
Who seem to know
My eyes are dim
and my wits are slow.
Blessed are they
That looked away
When coffee spilled
At the table today.
Blessed are they
With a cheery smile
Who stop to chat
For a little while.
Blessed are they
Who never say,
"You've told me that story
Twice today."
Blessed are they

Who know the ways
To bring back memories
Of yesterdays.
Blessed are they
Who make it known
That I'm loved, respected,
And not alone.
Blessed are they
Who know I'm at a loss
To find the strength
To carry the cross.
Blessed are they
Who ease the days
On my journey Home
In loving ways.

—Ester Mary Walker

Acknowledgements and Appreciation

To caregivers far and wide who have shared their stories,
dreams, poems, and spirit.

To Dorothy Bonnette for introducing me to so many
classic prayers and blessings.

To Tanya Looney for restoring her faith.

To Debra Medders for being a rock and a fortress.

To Sister Del Ray for doing the right thing and sharing it.

To the tender hearts of Countryside Place.

To Maureen Osis and Terry Bucher for rounding up such
grand material.

To Elise Nakhnikian of longermcareprovider.com where
some of these ideas first appeared.

To Share Ernst for moving beyond reaction to creation.

To Jill for saying "yes."

To Susan and the rest of the Hartman Family for moving
New Mexico next to Vermont.

To my students at Northern State Correctional Facility for
their honesty and inspiration.

To Dolly for keeping food in the house and dirt off the
floor while I wrote.

To my family who understood.

In some instances the names have been changed to avoid
heartache.

—Bethany Knight
Glover, Vermont, April 2001

January: Blessed are the poor in spirit, for theirs is the kingdom of heaven

Those who know the freedom of being poor in spirit speak of feeling blessed. Not motivated by greed or desire for great material wealth, they live life on a different plane, focusing on the joy of living, the majesty of relationships.

Caregivers who are poor in spirit see themselves as answering a call, not rationally weighing career options. While the world may consider them powerless, low on the totem pole, the humble caregiver approaches each day with a deep sense of security and certainty. She knows that her faith alone will preserve her in the midst of life's afflictions. She does not turn to her own resources nor rely on her achievements to overcome whatever difficulties she faces.

Such men and women are not peacocks pridefully displaying their feathers. Compliments are humbly received but do not falsely build egos. Leading lives of simplicity, they seem uninterested in flattery. Trusting in their God, their lives become the kingdom of heaven. If you're looking for someone to give you the shirt off her back, look no further.

A certified nursing assistant for 34 years, Mary Morrison had a full weekend planned when her employer summoned her to a national retreat in Atlanta. "You've been selected as a charter member of Mariner Post Acute Network Certified Nursing Assistant Professional Advisory Council."

"My son was getting out of prison, but I told him I had to go to Atlanta. I wanted to be on the Council," Mary recalled.

She was no stranger to having relatives in and out of prison. All three of her children were mentally handicapped, and trouble with the law came easily.

What caused the retardation? "Well," Mary would answer, "getting kicked in the stomach during every pregnancy, I expect."

A tiny woman with a fashion flair, Mary's eyes were deep and bright. Her hands were like leather gloves; how many thousands of times had she washed them while washing others?

Crowned Council Queen, Mary wrote her first poem:

> To me, caring means taking the time to love, listen and touch.
> To my residents these three things mean so much.
> Even if it is a second, a minute or an hour,
> These three things help my residents feel like they have power.
> If you're as afraid and fragile as they are
> This tells them that I'm their shining star.
> I am their family away from home
> When I care for my residents they never roam.
> I am the one they tell their stories to
> And I know that in the future it could be me or you.
> So when talking with my residents I'm not anxious
> Because I know caring is about being patient.
>
> —Love, Queen Mary
> Brian Center Health and Rehab, LaGrange, Georgia

TODAY *Shine like a star.*

Julia Jones walks through life like a woman on a free shopping spree at the grocery store. Everything looks interesting; she grabs a handful and keeps moving forward.

Julia has been a certified nursing assistant since she was a teenager. Now in her forties, there is little she hasn't mastered in a nursing home. Upon discovering that CPR classes were extraordinarily expensive, she became certified so she could offer them for $5 a person at her facility. She also took on staff scheduling, medical transport, orientation of new staff, drug testing, the nursing budget and more. When the activities director goes on vacation, Julia fills in. This is also true for covering vacancies in social services and rehabilitation.

One of life's cheerleaders, Julia doesn't roll with the punches, she just plain ignores them. When she decided to have a baby, 19 miscarriages preceded the birth of her treasured Jasmine.

Julia worked four jobs to give Jasmine a home, ballet lessons and after-school programs. Days off were unheard of, and Julia's only experience with sick days was filling in for others when they were ill.

Hearing about a new job at a brand-new facility, the curious Julia applied. Days later, she jubilantly celebrated her acceptance of a great offer.

"You know what the best part is? I can have just one job, and be like everyone else. Now I can volunteer at Jasmine's school, and help tutor kids in reading."

TODAY: *Prepare for your reward.*

Regardless of civilization or era, all communities of human beings have had activities and property that signal success, saying, "I made it."

During the first thousand years of recorded time in Europe, blessings from the dying and from caregivers were among the most sought-after possessions to receive. Both were seen as holy people: the dying because they had one foot in the next world, and the caregiver because she was humble.

Following a day-long workshop on caregiving held in a Wichita church, a group of nursing assistants was treated to a building tour and impromptu organ concert by the church organist. It was a powerful moment: 15 dedicated caregivers perched on pews, majestic music moving from the pipes to the vaulted ceilings. At times, the cushioned pews seemed to vibrate as the organ took over the sanctuary.

Afterwards, the CNAs were asked to stand and bless one another and all others present. The sacred nature of the gathering had not gone unnoticed.

Someone asked the organist, "Why do you play those constant really low notes?"

"That's the foundation of the piece; you can't have any music without it. Everything is based on them.... kind of like you, I suppose."

High quality nursing assistants are the foundation of all caregiving enterprises. Everything good is based on you.

TODAY: *Bless one another.*

To my cellist husband, the greatest composer who ever lived was Johann Sebastian Bach. Bach was a member of a remarkable family of musicians, whose three sons also became composers. J. S. Bach wrote all kinds of vocal and instrumental music, including the *Brandenburg Concertos*, the *Well-Tempered Clavier* and the *Mass in B minor*.

Like all great creators, Bach was inspired; he carried inside a Divine Spark. Certainly the study of music composition and learning to play instruments was essential to his success, but without his inner genius, nothing would have ever been produced.

Exceptional caregivers share Bach's deeply personal sense of inspiration. Of course, being well grounded and versed in the practice of caring for others is essential, but without one's heart as the motivator, the driving force, nothing enduring can be produced.

Whether he was writing a piece for the solo flute or a grand scale chorale for one hundred voices, Bach began each composition exactly the same way. Before one note was penned on to the blank sheet, he wrote his dedication on the upper-left-hand side of the page: To The Glory of God.

Summoning strength and a sense of mission at the beginning of every day, humble caregivers undoubtedly whisper a similar pledge.

TODAY: *Give glory where it is due.*

Entertainment Tonight blares the news of stars splitting and couples coupling. People magazine spills the nasty stories of celebrity addictions and rehab nightmares. We're forever being told about the diets, wardrobes and vacations of the rich and famous, whether we're interested or not.

With such constant reminders of their Bigness and our Smallness, what sense can we make of our own lives? No TV reporter seems interested in what we eat and wear, and our vacation spent cleaning the kids' rooms will hardly be broadcast by Mary Hart!

In truth, every life is just that, a full and complete life, worthy of right living and good works. Publicity and hype do not make a life better or more meaningful. In fact, how often do we hear the most popular singers and actors grieve for their privacy and a simple life when they are no longer able to go to the mall without being mobbed?

Your place of work, be it a hospital, nursing home, assisted living facility, school, group home or private home, is as rich and deserving as any Hollywood studio or mansion. Humanity is the great ocean, and your life is a single drop, containing all the ingredients of the ocean, just in a smaller amount. As you live, so could the world. Never minimize your greatness, your precious life and the gratitude of others for the gift that is you.

> To see a world in a grain of sand
> And heaven in a wild flower
> Hold infinity in the palm of your hand
> And eternity in an hour.

—William Blake, *Auguries of Innocence*

TODAY: *Hold infinity in the palm of your hand.*

From an advice column asking readers about doctors:

> Stand back. You're in the way of an avalanche. Doctors are motivated by greed..If you took the dollars out of medicine, our society would rid itself of the parasites in the medical field, as well as those in the pharmaceutical and insurance industries...these people are killing us...If I treated my clients the way doctors have treated me, I would be unemployed or in jail.

> Bob in Massachusetts

And from a Healthcare Provider Formerly Known as Doc:

> Government meddling, managed care, red tape and overzealous lawyers have totally destroyed the doctor-patient relationship. In the eyes of insurance companies, we are no longer physicians, but 'healthcare providers.' The rising cost of medicine has been a factor, but it is the MD who has taken the blame, even though our financial reimbursement has dropped substantially.

We've heard this and worse before. Americans no longer trust the healthcare system; they think it is expensive, poor in quality, and places too much emphasis on technology. Patients miss the bedside manner, the human touch, and the feeling that they matter.

Regardless of the extraneous and annoying pressures, humble caregivers who are poor in spirit don't take their eyes off the prize. Even when time is short, the human touch is always present.

TODAY: *Show that health care still has a human face.*

I Said a Prayer for You Today

I said a prayer for you today
And know God must have heard.
I felt the answer in my heart
Although He spoke not a word.
I didn't ask for wealth or fame
(I know you wouldn't mind).
I asked Him to send treasures
Of a far more lasting kind.
I prayed that He'd be near you
At the start of each new day,
To grant you health and blessings
And friends to share the way.
I asked for happiness for you
In all things great and small.
But it was for His loving care
I prayed the most of all.

—Anonymous

Today may be the birthday or anniversary date of a co-worker, or possibly the date s/he became a caregiver, some five or ten or more years ago. Perhaps someone in your care is celebrating today.

Rather than going to Wal-Mart, just go to the store of your heart—that storehouse of love and good will. You'll find whatever they need.

TODAY: *Say a prayer for someone.*

Since I live 20 miles from Canada, my mailbox is full of shopping guides and flyers, inviting me to cross the border and spend money to save money.

"What do you notice about this advertisement?" my husband asked one winter morning, handing me a full-color newsprint publication called *The Shopper: Your Saving Guide.*

Was it the prices? I didn't recognize a lot of the brands. Wait a minute.

"The grandmother in the picture!"

We both noticed her. The photograph was a kitchen table scene. Dad was leafing through *The Shopper,* with his son seated next to him, eagerly pointing to something. Standing to dad's right was a smiling mom. And standing to dad's left, looking over his shoulder sweetly, was GRANDMA!

How many times to do we see a healthy older woman in a commercial or business promotion? Rarely. Our older men and women are banished from the cameras, as Americans like to pretend we stay young and thin all our lives. Seeing Grandma in *The Shopper* made us happy, as the simple photo implied, "Our Grandma is still an important part of our life. She helps us make decisions and enjoy our home life together. She counts."

TODAY: *Value Grandmas.*

Perhaps more than anyone else, those blessed to be poor in spirit know the truth of the axiom, "It's the thought that counts."

My father specializes in garage sales, flea markets and other random dispersants of other people's junk. He loves a bargain and loves to shower his family with the bounty of his hunts.

For years I have collected hearts—on coffee mugs, jewelry, art, clothing, anything. Papa enjoys casting his net wide at sales in search of another heart. He's agreed to search for little heart pins I can use as favors and prizes during workshops and presentations.

During a particularly nasty Nor'easter, I flew as far as Boston before the airports closed. My home was one cancelled plane flight away. Closed runways left me deplaning at Logan's terminal E, the international gates, though I had only flown from Arkansas.

Hotels are routinely $150 a night or more in the Boston area, a charge I couldn't bear paying. Yet it was only 9:30 PM, and I couldn't face sitting up all night in the chilly terminal.

"$59.99 a night! Free shuttle!" the sign blinked, one of many designed to welcome foreigners to the States. I called and Kathy answered. She heard my anxiety and exhaustion and disappointment. I'd been gone two weeks, and I was missing home.

"We'll come and get you, don't worry," she promised, and sure enough, the van arrived and I was soon checking in. "Where's the candy machine? I didn't have any dinner and what I want is sweets—comfort food."

"We don't have one, I'm sorry," Kathy said, "But wait."

From under the counter she pulled a basket of European chocolates, wrapped in Christmas foils. She gave me a big handful. I felt so cared for!

The next morning, I left a thank-you note with the day clerk for Kathy, and attached one of my dad's heart stickpins.

"Dear Mrs. Knight: I am writing to say thank you for your wonderful gift. The pin is really lovely and will be worn every day." Kathy mailed me a note that week, and closed hoping we would meet again one day.

TODAY: *Please pass the hearts.*

For more than 30 years, the nursing home world has been defined and designed by government. Staff training, resident quality indicators and environmental conditions are dictated by those who do not live or work in nursing homes. Some observers suggest that having care defined by individuals who prefer to sit at desks and write rules rather than provide care is the cruelest twist of fate yet.

Consequently, a very real piece of a human being's experience of life, his spiritual life, can remain virtually unnamed and unimportant in the eyes of regulators and surveyors. Caregivers can unknowingly surrender their sense of spirit by losing perspective and becoming obsessed by the government's power and unannounced inspections.

Our challenge daily, in the midst of the sterile environment outlined by policies and protocols, is to see the extraordinary in the ordinary. With this set of eyes, we quickly recognize that repositioning a patient every two hours through the night is not just to be in compliance with the law, or even to prevent bedsores. Rather, this wordless moment of tenderness is loving reassurance in the dark of night, reminding residents they are not alone.

With this set of eyes, we quickly recognize that changing an adult incontinent product is not just to keep someone dry and comfortable, but may well be the longest period of contact they have with another human being all day. And even the simple act of washing a window becomes an opportunity to create a clear view of the world beyond.

Out of this awareness, you can discover the significance of your work and see the impact of your contribution. Through the performance of ordinary daily tasks you can define and honor the spiritual life of your facility.

TODAY: *See the extraordinary in the ordinary.*

Oh, I used to love snow days. Just think: Mother Nature loved me so much that she would pile snow high enough during the night to force the cancellation of school. Wow.

When my son Elliot was little, he would bring that same sleepy excitement to the radio on icy mornings, hoping against hope to hear "Montpelier Elementary is closed." Surrounding country school districts would always close, the roads being too risky for bus travel. But the city rarely had to close school, and Elliot came to feel discriminated against. He begged that we move out of town.

I couldn't blame him. We all feel hemmed in and overly managed by city life. The more man is able to control the environment, the less mystery life holds.

Now I do live in the country, and I still love snow days. We have a glass barometer full of turquoise-colored water, and when the water starts to climb the stem, it means a front is coming through. Yippee, an Act of God! The power goes out and we cook on the woodstove, use candles, listen to our crank radio, watch the barometer and thermometer and somehow, in experiencing the unknown, we feel safer. Back to basics, keep it simple, focus on the quiet between us. Cut loose from our phones, computers and television, we are blessed to be poor in spirit.

Caregivers who live in four season climates are well acquainted with the contingency plans triggered by Acts of God. Doug, a darling CNA at Countryside Place in Mishawaka, Indiana recalled the valiant efforts of his coworkers during a fierce winter storm. "They were amazing. They were ready to sleep here, work double shifts, help in the kitchen, whatever was needed."

Crises call forth our best. Next time there's an Act of God, watch how you act like God.

TODAY: *Act like God.*

Growing up in the United States, we are trained from an early age to identify and solve problems.

Remember story problems in math class? Those darn 35-gallon fish bowls and how much water five four-ounce angelfish would displace? (I always wondered why anyone would need to figure this out. Wouldn't you take some water out if needed when you added the fish? Sheesh.)

Women's magazines and television programs are full of makeovers, with before pictures of poor ugly ducklings who, voila! are transformed by Leo of Hollywood and his 15-person crew. In America, everything and everyone is a candidate to be improved, a problem to be solved, enhanced, fixed by cosmetic surgery.

Living in India my 18th summer, I was stunned by the absence of this problem/solution mentality. People didn't walk around proposing improvements. And when something did come up, like flies landing on the food, they did something that left my Western head spinning: they put a dish of sugar on the table for the flies, and the flies complied.

As I have aged and fallen deeply in love with India and its people, I have learned about maya, the Hindu belief that all we see is illusion and what is real is what can't be seen. Squabbles, troubles and problems are just distractions, keeping one from a real-life relationship with the Universal Self, the great love that unites us all. Grounded in the eternal, Hindus ignore the fleeting annoyances of the material world. All is maya.

TODAY: *Get grounded in the eternal.*

Used bookstores are full of stories. The stories aren't just on the pages of the books, but on the envelopes, photos, postcards and other scraps of paper that once served as bookmarks.

Virtually every tiny town I visited in Ireland had its own used bookstore. Browsing through the hardback novels in the little store in Dalkey, I found and bought the sequel to *Gone with the Wind.* In Ireland? Reading the book, I learned Scarlett O'Hara returns to her Irish roots, and even survives the famine.

The book also offered up a frayed strip of cardboard with this blessing:

> Let nothing disturb thee.
> Let nothing affright thee.
> All things are passing.
> God never changes.
> Patience gains all things.
> Who has God wants nothing.
> God alone suffers.

Like finding money or a four-leaf clover, there is something magical, even mystical, about a stranger's message fluttering from a book. What is the Universe trying to tell me? What am I supposed to learn?

Traveling by myself, I took great comfort in my bookmark's promises. The random nature of the blessing affirmed my belief that I am never alone, regardless of where I am or what I am doing. I need not be afraid. I am safe. I am loved.

TODAY: *Look and listen for unexpected blessings.*

A Call From God

Although I am not extremely religious, I do believe in God.

When I was 17, I started helping the elderly. This would be my journey through life. I worked in a little townhouse taking care of seven people at night. The lady I worked with took people right into her home.

Yes, she was a loving, caring person on a crusade! I worked there at night so she could sleep, only to get up the next morning to serve these loved ones.

I worked in two other places before moving on to the best place I have ever worked, Maple Lane in Barton, Vermont. Yes, the building is nice but that's not going to do the work for these beautiful people we care for every day. We are the hands that feed them, and the legs that help them walk. God bless these people. They did not ask to end up this way.

So, if you're in it for the money, you better leave. That's not what a true nurses' aide cares about. Yes, there are times that you might get mad, and it takes a lot of patience. You don't make a lot of money, but the smiles on their faces should be enough reward for you! Yes, I've gotten mad at doing someone else's work, too, but I feel that everyone is there to do his or her own job. Yes, you get upset if you're hit, scratched or kicked.

I guess the bottom line is I don't think they asked God to make them this way. I don't think they said, "Well, when I get old I'm going to hit these aides." They didn't ask to be this way and we won't either. We are all coming to this, and patience is indeed a virtue. You see you don't get love and thanks from one patient. You receive it from many.

This word "caring" makes a true nurses' aide. But everyone in a nursing home should be honored, for all of them bring love to these special people. Housekeeping cleans their room like they were able to clean their houses before. Laundry does their clothes for they no longer can do for themselves. Kitchen makes their meals so they may eat. I'm sure they wish they could still prepare their own.

Office takes care of their business, so they no longer have to worry about anything. Administration and activities make their lives more comfortable for them, to live day by day. Daycare takes care of the staff's little ones. All departments bring their hearts full of love, to many people, everyday.

—Rhonda Monfette
Rhonda has worked as a nursing assistant for 32 years, well over half her life.

TODAY: *Bring your heart full of love.*

The old circus elephant looked like she was nearing the end of her tour. Welts, scars, bumps and dents marked Daisy's toughened hide, souvenirs of countless parades and performances.

We're like Daisy, toting around the damage unfairly inflicted upon us during our journey. Fifth grade gym class, being the last one picked for the kickball squad. Ninth grade dance, never asked to Twist. Age 30, overhearing coworkers gossiping about me. My wounds may not be as visible as Daisy's, but these stored memories are with me, dangerously shaping my reactions and actions in a brand new day.

If I am to live as one who is poor in spirit, I cannot rely upon yesterday's baggage for guidance. Hauling the past into the present only guarantees one outcome: reliving my pain. Instead, I have come to think of my memories as stored mass I must discard. Like a log tossed into the fire, the past provides me energy for today. Processing and working through painful recollections, I grow and move forward.

Mass is the substance of the created universe, the matter that makes the earth. What stored mass is fueling you? Daily discarding of old hurts gives us more energy for the present. As my Grandma Tante used to say when cleaning a closet, "If in doubt, throw it out!"

TODAY: *Let go.*

Just when my family thought they knew me, I mastered the headstand. Age 48, with gravity taking its toll, I stuck my toes into the sky.

I've longed to be someone who could do a headstand since my cabinmate flipped up into one at Girl Scout camp. Headstands came to symbolize freedom, breaking the rules, being independent. To snap into a headstand would mean I had a carefree spirit, untethered by convention. Oh, I wanted to do a headstand.

Unfortunately, I brought equally intense feelings to the fear that held my feet on terra firma: I was afraid I would break my neck. I suppose someone once relayed a story of someone who had become paralyzed attempting a headstand.

Like my experience driving a go-cart, I floored the brake and the accelerator at the same time and froze.

Melissa, my yoga teacher, replaced my blind anxiety with her calming instruction. Breaking a headstand into many steps, she showed me how to slowly balance my weight on three points, tipping myself gradually and methodically until the headstand almost happened by itself. I cried victory and declared a new family holiday the day I went up and down without being next to a wall.

Confronting and disposing of fear is a mighty way to build one's self-confidence and trust. My headstands have greatly influenced my overall sense of worth. I learned I could count on myself, that I won't let myself down. I learned that I could call upon an inner strength greater than my fears.

TODAY: *Call upon inner strength.*

Joan Chittister writes:

> Our entire generation has gone deaf. Scripture and wisdom and relationships and personal experience are all being ignored. We are, consequently, a generation of four wars and of the most massive arms buildup in the history of the world, in a period called peacetime. We are a generation of great poverty in the midst of great wealth, of great loneliness in the center of great communities; of serious personal breakdowns and community deterioration in the face of unparalleled social growth....We believe in action and results and products and profit and youth, so we come to regard the elderly as essentially useless.

Do you long for the good old days?

An old friend used to complain about any number of societal ills by opening his comments with the same phrase, "Nowadays..." I would laugh, wondering how a 25-year-old had such a long frame of reference. Had the world changed so much in his short lifetime?

Tonight while I made dinner, two situation comedies played on TV. Obviously, lots of kids were watching as their parents prepared the meal. Both shows included plot lines that alluded to male characters having less than adequate genitals. Too small.

What were little kids in the audience thinking, I wondered? Why do we feel such silliness is worth featuring on a family show? I was sad and angry, thinking my own "nowadays" thoughts.

I was reminded of Joan Chittister's words about "community deterioration." As professionals whose lives are about not ignoring relationships, personal experience and the elderly, we must uphold the standards of civility and grace. Leading by example, caregivers remind the world that life is precious, holy and worthy of great regard.

TODAY: *Uphold the standards of civility and grace.*

My friend George lives in Thunder Bay, Ontario, Canada. He jokes that he can tell when his neighbors have had a fight: "The UPS trucks start to arrive with the 'I deserve this because you owe me' packages."

One-click online ordering and gorgeous direct mail catalogues that arrive by the dozen make shopping too easy. I remember hearing a woman say she wouldn't order anything that doesn't arrive within three days. "When it comes much later, I don't even know why I ordered it."

Buying pretty things is fun. So is finding perfect presents for friends. But it can be an exhausting avocation.

One of the many grand yet unanticipated gifts of my October 2000 trip to Ireland was that I couldn't shop. Not for any noble reasons. I just had a small suitcase that had to stay small so I could carry it on flights.

Part of my stay included a personal retreat on the Irish Sea, at St. Teresa's, a Carmelite convent. On her day off, Sister Francis offered to take me by subway into Dublin. Our walking tour included churches, a café, and yes, the Pound Store. Just like the Dollar Store "in the colonies," the Pound Store was loaded with cute, inexpensive wares made by the Chinese.

For a split second, I privately pouted that I didn't have room in my suitcase to fit an adorable straw hat. Then, suddenly, I felt helium-filled. "I can't buy anything!" I told Sister, "and it's fine!"

I didn't have to worry about whether it was a good price, if I should comparison shop, if I really needed it, where I would put it, if it was the right size and color or what my husband would say. I just browsed and enjoyed Sister's company. I felt happier than I could remember on any shopping trip.

TODAY: *Stop shopping!*

Prior to the life of Christ, caring for the sick was a job for families only. The Romans left sick paupers lying on the roadside, believing their families didn't regard them as worth saving. Only three kinds of people were rescued because of their value to the economy: soldiers, gladiators and slaves.

Society's values toward the poor were transformed by the life of Christ, ending the acceptability of human road kill. Believing Jesus might return any day, in disguise and possibly as a sick person, Christians regarded caregiving as holy work. All of one's shortcomings and mistakes could be absolved by caring for others.

Pilgrims walking to the Holy Land through the Alps became the first patients, falling ill far from their families. Usually taking the journey as a form a penance or for healing, pilgrims were already in a weakened condition. Travel was tough, the food strange and insufficient. Monasteries opened up hospices and infirmaries to serve the sick pilgrims, with priests and nuns the earliest caregivers.

In Syria in 370 AD, St. Basil opened his hospital and leprosarium. About one hundred years later, also in Syria, the Hospice of Turmanin was built as a campus, and included a church, an office building, a convent and the inn for dispensing hospitality to pilgrims.

By the year 1000 in Cluny, France, monasteries were building open wards in the shape of the cross, believing the design would aid healing. In the center was a chapel and altar visible to all patients, where daily communion was served. The layout also aided ventilation and supervision.

With the Reformation, care of the sick and operation of hospitals was taken from the Church and assumed by the King. The Crown began to collect taxes to support care of the poor, creating Europe's first system of social aid.

An order was issued in London in 1569 that the aged, sick, lame or blind shall be sent to St. Bartholomew's or St. Thomas's hospitals, as admission depended one's town of residence. By the 18th Century, it became too complicated to send sick people to the hospital nearest their original parish. The new, nondiscriminating admissions policy: "Whatever corner of the world they come from they come without restriction," also became the foundation of the American hospital movement. The first hospitals built in the New World were Pennsylvania Hospital in Philadelphia, Massachusetts General in Boston and New York Hospital in New York City.

Healthcare providers of today are linked to this rich history. The wings built off a central area in modern nursing homes and hospitals are direct descendants of the ancient cross design. And like the caregivers of old, you are still called to perform holy work, to care when families are no longer able.

TODAY: *Perform holy work.*

Being a nurses' aide means caring, sharing, loving and understanding. To always be there with open hands, to assist in every way you can. Communicating with your patient is important so they know they are still loved and not abandoned during this time of illness.

You must understand that your patients are people just like you are and not just a number. They may be old and contracted and maybe can't see or hear, but they, too, are made of flesh and blood and have feelings.

Just remember one thing, my fellow classmates, as one day this was said to me: "As you care for your patients, take a look at your hands and think to yourself, these are the kind of hands I want to take care of me, if ever I should be as helpless and alone."

These people did not choose to be where they are, but you, the nurses' aide, have the choice to be where you are.

This is not just a job; this is a very fulfilling and rewarding commitment. It takes a very special person to be a nurses' aide, and I feel I am one of them.

—Written for recently certified nursing assistants by Debbie Salerno, a CNA at Mountainview Care Center, Scranton, Pennsylvania

TODAY: *Be there with open hands.*

Author Helen M. Luke writes:

> No, the sickness of our society is not due to the threat of the bomb, the ineptitude or corruption of the Establishment, to wars or to the machinations of Communists or Capitalists. These evils are effects, not causes; they have always existed and are no worse because of the enormous scale on which they now operate.
>
> Our sickness is fundamentally due to the breakdown of the symbolic life which all the great religions have existed to maintain, so that we are left with eyes that see not and ears that hear not beyond the literal facts and voice of our environment. We hear only the dark news of the broadcaster and our inner ear is deaf to the song of angels.

The dark news of the broadcasters can be heard 24 hours a day, with international atrocities and tragedies repeated on the hour. But where do we go to hear the Song of Angels?

Where do children go to see good works being done in their community? Where can cynics see that people really are good at heart? Where do frail elders depend on the kindness of strangers?

All roads lead to you. Where two or more caregivers are gathered, we can hear the Song of Angels. But too often caregivers shy away from singing, convinced their lives are not worthy of song: "I'm nobody special; I don't have anything to share."

How wrong you are. In truth, your songs are music for our hearts, the healing balm that can cure what ails us. For the sake of our national soul, please, break your silence. All life will be treasured, and peace will comfort the planet, when the caregivers of the world tell their precious love stories.

TODAY: *Sing the song of angels.*

(Reprinted with the permission of Parabola Books, New York, www.parabola.org, from *Dark Wood to White Rose* by Helen Luke. Copyright © 1989. Appeared in Introduction, p. XIV).

While we're busy worrying we'll be late for work or that the rent check will bounce, our hearts stay on task, beating thousands of times daily and pumping five million gallons of blood in a lifetime.

That is, unless the arteries become blocked with fat and cause a heart attack, a leading killer in the U.S.

Blocked arteries routinely lead to bypass surgery, where the surgeon sews a new piece of blood vessel to bridge over or bypass the blockage. If the surgeon repairs three of the arteries it is called a triple bypass; four arteries, a quadruple bypass. The blood vessel used to create the bypass is taken from the chest or the leg.

Coronary artery bypass surgery provides detours around the partially or completely blocked arteries to improve a person's quality of life. Of course blockages and heart attacks can be prevented by not smoking, avoiding salt, maintaining a low-cholesterol diet, controlling blood pressure and getting regular exercise.

The routine and popular nature of heart bypass surgery is a metaphor for American life. Rather than acknowledging the precious quality of our lives, and the proper care and feeding we all deserve, Americans simply detour their hearts. If only we would live as we were designed to live! As a muscle and reservoir of love, the heart is the true keeper of the Divine Spark. It surely deserves the tenderest loving care.

TODAY: *Care for your heart.*

So, since January 15 you've been thinking about letting go. But how?

Thomas Keating, a Cistercian priest, suggests practicing contemplative prayer:

> When you practice contemplative prayer on a regular basis, your natural resources for psychic health begin to revive and you see the false value systems that are damaging your life. The emotional programs of early childhood that are buried in your unconscious begin to emerge into clear and stark awareness....expelling chunks of emotional junk. The principle discipline of contemplative prayer is letting go.

Eastern and Western religious traditions include the practice of contemplative prayer, sometimes referred to as meditation. Seeking quiet, we can begin to pay attention to our inner life, to that singular voice within.

At a workshop hosted by Zen Buddhist priest Norman Fisher of the San Francisco Zen Center, we discussed meditation as an antidote to consumerism. "Consumerism is the further evolution of capitalism," Fisher told us. We have become confused about what we need and want, the necessities versus the extras. Without spending time in contemplative prayer, we remain on the surface, settling for activities that cater to sensual pleasures, which do not last.

By simply pausing and withdrawing from the daily circus, we can regain our sense of balance and purpose, rejoicing in the blessing that comes from being poor in spirit.

TODAY: *Take time to contemplate.*

(Reprinted from *Open Mind, Open Heart, The Contemplative Dimension of the Gospel* by Thomas Keating. Copyright © 1998. The Continuum International Publishing Group. Reprinted with permission from the publisher.)

Caregivers are underpaid because the citizens of the United States of America haven't recognized the value of care. We're talking about priorities. And to think our nation's present priorities are what they should be is a naïve mistake.

Priorities evolve over generations because courageous people speak up, and speak up, and speak up.

In 1909, the U.S. Bureau of Animal Husbandry, within the Department of Agriculture, had a staff of more than 1,000 and a budget of $1.25 million.

> Far more money was spent each year on animal research than on research into the problems of early childhood—and as a result, the mortality rate of young animals was lower than that of young children.

President Herbert Hoover believed providing public relief to the poor was not the job of the federal government.

> Hoover's attitude was exemplified in 1930, when he approved a congressional appropriation of $45 million to feed stricken livestock of Arkansas farmers but opposed an additional $25 million to feed starving farmers and their families.

Fortunately, compassionate and vocal citizens rallied, organized and lobbied for federal aid to the poor.

Today, united voices are needed to call for a national reverence for life, and particularly the life of the very young and very old. These vulnerable populations deserve our utmost respect and resources, as do those who are devoted to providing them vital care.

TODAY: *Speak up for your priorities.*

(Reprinted with the permission of The Free Press, a Division of Simon & Schuster, Inc., from *From Poor Law to Welfare State: A History of Social Welfare in America* by Walter I. Trattner. Copyright © 1974, 1979, 1984, 1989 by The Free Press. Copyright © 1994, 1998 by Walter I. Trattner.)

Society looks to religiously sponsored nonprofit institutions, such as hospitals and nursing homes, to model the highest standard of employer-employee relations.

The National Interfaith Committee for Worker Justice offers a code of conduct booklet to help union leadership and healthcare management understand one another, communicate respectfully and build healthy working relationships.

The 10-page booklet, *Guidelines for Unions and Management of Religiously Sponsored Health Care Institutions*, was developed in the midst of great change and tension in the healthcare industry.

"There is an increase in religion-labor organizing efforts in the healthcare industry to secure a voice, living wages, better benefits, job security, respect, and fairness in the workplace," said Bishop Jesse DeWitt, retired from the United Methodist Church and president of the National Interfaith Committee's board.

"Our hope is that this document will be widely used as a tool for reflection, dialogue and relationship building," said Sister Barbara Pfarr, SSND, Religious Employer Project Coordinator for the Interfaith Committee. "We believe these rules of engagement are a concrete contribution towards finding solutions to a longstanding problem."

The Chicago-based National Interfaith Committee educates, organizes, and mobilizes the religious community in the U.S. on issues and campaigns that will improve wages, benefits, and working conditions for workers, especially low-wage workers.

TODAY: *Foster healthy working relationships.*

Preparing for holiday visitors, I decided it was time to clean the drawers and cupboard under the sink in our guest bathroom. I use the bathroom when we don't have company, leaving my husband the other upstairs bath, what I call "the boys' bathroom."

Pawing through leaking, dried-out or otherwise useless tubes and vials of cosmetics and hair care potions, I can't believe what I have accumulated. How many half-empty masks, facial scrubs and apricot peels have I tried? There are at least as many astringents, all promising clearer, cleaner skin and smaller pores. The truth is, I got my Grandpa Timothy Purcell's big pores, and nothing shrinks them. But I keep buying whatever is new, expecting a miracle.

Have I been so insecure over the past 15 years that I really believed well-being could be found in a magic bottle? What was I thinking? I have an equally crowded and untouched shelf of diet books, recipes and weight-loss plans. More instant remedies.

Beyond the neediness and lack of self-confidence these purchases reveal, I see how I have wasted money that could have made a difference in someone else's life. Even lipstick is at least $5. How many children could I feed and clothe with my hair-conditioning budget?

What do you buy that you don't need? To feel and look truly beautiful, we need to listen to that insecure girl inside, and remind her she is loved. Blessed are the poor in spirit.

TODAY: *Listen to the insecure one inside.*

I save the fortunes from fortune cookies and tape them on my radio: Sell your ideas—they are totally acceptable. Meeting adversity well is the source of your strength. You are going to have a very comfortable old age. Stop searching forever; happiness is just next to you. Many receive advice, only the wise profit from it. Love or fame, you'll be able to handle either or both. Long life is in store for you.

Call me silly, but my cookie fortunes are a source of great inspiration and hope.

I am fascinated by the Chinese culture, particularly the delicate art. Our culture is embryonic in comparison. In fact, the Chinese calendar is the longest chronological record in history, dating from 2600 BC. The Chinese see time in 60-year segments of five 12-year cycles. Thus, the year 2001 and 1989 are both the Year of the Snake.

The Chinese Lunar Calendar names each of the 12 years after an animal. Legend has it that the Lord Buddha summoned all the animals to come to him before he departed from earth. Only 12 came to bid him farewell and as a reward he named a year after each one in the order they arrived. The Chinese believe the animal ruling the year in which a person is born has a profound influence on personality, saying: "This is the animal that hides in your heart." (I'm a Dragon!)

Because the lunar calendar is based on the cycles of the moon, the beginning of the year can fall anywhere between late January and the middle of February. Families and friends visit one another during the first two weeks of the New Year, and enjoy a variety of lucky foods. Among the luckiest are peanuts, called Zao, said to promote longevity.

Why not stop at the grocery store on the way to work today and pick up a bag of peanuts in the shell? Put a bowl in the break room and wish everyone Happy New Year and a long life!

TODAY: *Wish everyone a long life.*

George Washington Carver was a genius inventor who lived from 1864 to 1943.

Born a slave, he devoted much of his life to teaching and research at the Tuskegee Institute in Alabama. We know him for his in-depth study of the peanut and what it could produce. Carver believed peanuts could meet almost every need. His life work included developing—from peanuts—flour, meal, bird food, milk, a sauce comparable to soy sauce, cheese, a coffee-like drink, ink and more.

We know less of Carver the man, and that is our loss. A spiritual, humble and frugal man who had no children of his own, he was forever dispensing advice to students, whom he loved as family.

This is from a letter dated January 9, 1922 from Carver to a member of the Tuskegee senior class.

> Possession of these eight cardinal virtues constitutes a lady or a gentleman:
>
> Be clean both inside and out.
> Who neither looks up to the rich nor down on the poor.
> Who loses, if need be, without squealing.
> Who wins without bragging.
> Who is always considerate of women, children and old people.
> Who is too brave to lie.
> Who is too generous to cheat.
> Who takes his share of the world and lets other people have theirs.

TODAY: *Practice Carver's eight virtues.*

(Reprinted from *George Washington Carver: In His Own Words*. Edited by Gary R. Kremer, by permission of the University of Missouri Press. Copyright © 1987 by the Curators of the University of Missouri.)

Experience is always our best teacher, though some experiences aren't pleasant.

Such is often the case for families who have a relative needing long-term care. Usually a fall or some other incident sends a loved one to the hospital. Pressured by a reduction in Medicare funds, the hospital works to get the patient discharged as soon as possible. In my mother-in-law Frances' case last fall, the hospital sent her home at three in the morning with sky-rocketing blood pressure. I was outraged by this decision, particularly since she lives alone.

For those individuals who go directly from the hospital to the nursing home, discharge can be just as irrational. Based on payment rules, hospitals try to move patients early in the day, so the money received for providing care doesn't have to be spent on the patient. What a sick incentive. (pun intended!)

To the frightened soul who wants to go home, there is an expectation that the hospital and nursing home and home health personnel and physician are all talking to one another, that they all look at the same records—a most logical expectation, but rarely what happens.

Each provider group is privately operated and owned, with separate rules, budgets and staff. After a patient completes a successful stay in a nursing home for rehabilitation following a stroke, she is discharged home. Wouldn't it make sense to have the physical and occupational and speech therapists who treat her in the nursing home follow her home? Wouldn't it be nice to have those who help her relearn how to walk up stairs and open a jar actually see her master these tasks? In Vermont, such a logical follow-through by medical professionals is illegal, because nursing homes cannot be licensed to provide even limited home health services. So the patient must begin again with a new group of therapists, and, yes, be fully reevaluated (with Medicare billed). Most patients are confused and upset by these rules—anxiety they surely don't need.

Such rules protect provider turf but do little to promote continuity of care. Until medicine in America is truly designed and operated with patients at the center of decisions, such inefficient foolishness will continue. A pity.

TODAY: *Ease your patients' transfer anxiety.*

For more than 15 years, I have been the guardian of one or two of the elderly Coburn sisters. First I had younger sister Florence as my ward. Florence asked me to find her sister, Julia, who in turn asked if I would be her guardian. Florence died in 1998, so it's just Julia and me now.

Last autumn, Julia began to fall and became more confused. She needed nursing home care. Like all families, I had hoped Julia could avoid this day, and have her years end peacefully where she had been living. Her move was further complicated by my trip to Ireland. Thanks to the incredible attentions of Tina Donahue of the Central Vermont Council on Aging and Betty Blouin of Project Independence of Barre, Vermont, Julia's move to Union House Nursing Home was smooth. Returning to the states, I spent time with Julia, meeting her new roommate and caregivers.

We were so blessed! Not only were Julia and roommate Jean compatible, but Julia loved her nursing assistants, particularly Tausha. A tiny, sweet mother of four daughters, Tausha loved Julia from day one, and the feeling was obviously mutual. I was thrilled to see them together, touching each other's arms, little kisses passed. Thank you, God, for this wonderful arrangement.

With Christmas coming, I wanted to do something for this single mother, the light of Julia's life. Could I buy some presents for her children? Clothing? Food? How about a meal out and a movie?

"Oh, no," Tausha told me. "We can't take anything like that. I wouldn't feel right. I already get paid."

I had to respect her wishes, though I longed to personally acknowledge the care she provided Julia. My little compromise was to have Julia hand out gifts to staff members, including some cozy flannel pajamas to Tausha.

But oh, how I wanted to give Tausha the moon!

TODAY: *Realize how much families appreciate you.*

Today is my son Elliot's birthday. On this day in 1980 I became a mom, and began a wonderful adventure with this very cool person. After 27 hours of labor, my doctor decided to sit me on a birthing chair and let gravity help this boy find his way out.

The chair seat was horseshoe-shaped. A mirror was placed on the floor. I continued to push and looked into the mirror. Suddenly, a little face with black shiny eyes stared back at me. He looked like he was peaking through a hole in the fence!

"Take my glasses. I don't want to see anymore or I'll just stare and forget to push," I said.

I was a lucky mother, being the first to see my baby's face. The laws of physics usually prohibit this!

My face was the first of millions Elliot will see in his lifetime. I sometimes wonder, "Who will be the last?"

Mothers throughout time and round the world have wondered the same thing. We all hope and pray that final face is a loving and tender one, a kind set of eyes and hands providing comfort and reassurance. Every human being deserves such a grace-filled goodbye.

Yours may well be the last face, the last voice in a patient's precious life. Your name could be the last on his lips.

TODAY: *Give grace-filled goodbyes.*

February: Blessed are those who mourn, for they shall be comforted.

Mourning is typically associated with the death of a loved one, but we can mourn or grieve over the loss of a variety of things held dear: health, independence, youth, privacy, wealth, relationships, a sense of purpose.

Though little of life is predictable, we can be certain that the older we get, the more loss we will face. Moving from one neighborhood or town to another, seeing a favorite coach or pastor take another job, or suffering the accidental death of a family pet are fairly early experiences of loss that lead to mourning.

Some of us see the loosening of societal morals and standards as cause for great grief. We worry about the increased presence of guns in our communities and homes. A child is killed by a gun every two hours in the United States. We are all the bereaved here, mourning the loss of children and innocence, as well as our collective sense of safety.

One in five children in our country of 13.5 million live in poverty; 160 million children go hungry around the globe. We bemoan and mourn world affairs and our seeming inability to use the planet's great technology and wealth to feed children.

Caregivers are forever making sacrifices and facing loss. Fragile individuals in our care are often nursing broken hearts brought on by life's abrupt changes and endings. The challenge to all who mourn is to get beyond the injustice, pain or cruelty, accept sorrow and learn from it. In turn, the Beatitude promises comfort now.

Can we really expect or receive immediate comfort?

Thanks to the abundance of Universal Love, days are blessed with split-second moments that fill our hearts with healing. The glance of another, a sunset, a kitten pouncing across the floor...we only need look about and the comfort abounds.

Telling strangers our troubles is often easier than talking with friends. I find this to be especially true on beaches and on trips by train, plane or bus.

Bobbie worked in California's Silicon Valley. We landed next to each other on a day-long bus tour in Northern Ireland, neither of us with a traveling companion. I liked her immediately.

Talking about the dangers involved with one's spouse working on a household project "unsupervised," she tickled me with the question, "Why do men put thermostats right in the middle of a perfectly good wall?"

In the course of the day we moved way beyond jokes and swapping reading lists. I shared some of the uncertainties related to being self-employed; she dispelled the myths of job security in the high-tech world. Trusting her judgment and healthy outlook, I shared a deeply personal and painful event. "What can I do about it?" I asked her. "It is such a mess and I don't know how to get out of it."

Bobbie talked to me about the purpose of dark times in our lives, about seeing such moments as an encounter with the presence of evil, of Darkness itself. "Bethany, when you are in the dark, and the tiniest pin-prick of light appears, aren't your eyes drawn to that? Well, you are that light. And the Darkness wants to swallow you up, because you keep things from being dark and bleak. Don't let it get to you. Keep being that bright light."

A wave of relief and comfort ran through me. I was immediately quieted and at peace. I let go of my fear and anger and regained my sense of worth and control over my life.

TODAY: *Comfort a new friend.*

I attended an all-day meeting in Kansas City with other CNAs and learned I wasn't the only one who had problems with all the different hats a CNA puts on in the course of a day taking care of the elderly. Bethany made me realize what we do as CNAs is not a job but a career and we need to be professional in what we do.

I returned to work where I am one of the "regulars" (as the residents call me) who work in the Medicare wing. I was doing my daily duties on that hall and Mary called me into her room. She asked if I could help her to the restroom and then put her to bed.

After returning to her room and putting her down for a nap, I gave her a little kiss. Mary said, "Thank you" and I had to ask "Why?"

Mary told me with a tear in her eye that she missed the old me. "What do you mean 'the old me'?" I asked.

"Every time you put me to bed, you always used to give me a kiss on the cheek and say, 'Sleep well.' You have not done that in so long and I have looked forward to it every day," she said.

Now that both of us were in tears I asked, "Are you the only one I do this with?" and she said, "No! You used to do it with everyone and we all love the way you love us."

Now every day I go to work I am reminded of what Mary told me that day. I try to remember it all day so that I will not lose my way down the path of being the best CNA I can be to everyone that I care for.

I believe the moral of the story is that all of our residents, no matter how mobile or verbal, still love to be loved by their CNAs. Remember: it is not the facility that we work for, it's the people that we work with. And that is why I am a CNA.

—Lisa Yoakum, CNA, works at
Beverly Healthcare in Pittsburg, Kansas

TODAY: *Comfort those you work for.*

Have you met one of these troubled families? Unable to properly care for mom at home, they come to you expecting perfect days, never a mistake and sometimes even miracles.

"She should never wear any clothing with food stains!"

"Why hasn't my mother seen the doctor yet?"

While these sons and daughters have decided they cannot handle taking care of mom or dad at home, they expect nursing home staff to have no difficulty in doing so. Complaining about care is how they show they care. And the louder they complain, the more they believe they care.

It is always smart to keep these facts in mind and not take any complaints seriously. Caregivers also need to understand that we are a culture afraid of aging and death. When we must move a parent to a nursing home, we feel guilty. We think, "I should be able to care for her myself!"

Guilt allows us to believe we care without taking any action.

Families need to be taught there is no reason to fear age or death, and that caregivers can deal tenderly and lovingly with their loved ones. As you talk with visiting relatives, strive to convey the natural aspects of this phase of life in small and gentle ways. Conversations about spiritual subjects are usually delicate but often very welcome. It may be that these grieving sons and daughters can only talk to you. Yes, their mom or dad is failing, but this only makes memories more precious and important. Be open to questions and cues, and seek to bring comfort.

TODAY: *Comfort troubled families.*

In *Death of a Hired Man*, poet Robert Frost wrote that "Home is where, when you have to go there, they have to take you in." The poem tells the tale of a former employee returning to a couple he had worked for and who had let him go. Gradually it becomes clear to Mary and Warren that Silas has come home to die.

As a child, on cold winter weekends I would put my blanket and pillow over the floor vent near the picture window and be warmed by the furnace and the sun. The wind-up clock lulled me to sleep. Decades later, napping beside a different sunny picture window and heating grate, another old clock ticks me to sleep. My eyes closed, I am a child again in my parents' home.

To be close to the familiar feels good. I have heard stories of old farmers living in nursing homes who wander out into the long grasses, curl up on the ground and die.

Nothing about the institutional surroundings is familiar to your residents. And yet they have the same longings as the hired man or the old farmers—a desire to be known and comforted by the known. Caregivers in such circumstances are asked to offer hospitality to a stranger. By providing tender loving care the caregiver creates a comforting atmosphere. No, the walls are not familiar. But the quality of your kindness can awaken a memory, perhaps of another time, far away, when care was given.

Listening to grief, offering sympathy and managing your patients' pain are your charge. While they may come from a world very different from yours, life's common human denominators link you together.

TODAY: *Comfort strangers.*

Marlene is not exactly comfortable with death, but she is no longer squeamish either. Caring for others for more than 20 years, she has made peace with the sudden appearance of death. Told by supervisors to avoid grief by not getting close to her patients, Marlene consciously chose to ignore the advice. "If I don't get close to them, what's the point of caring for them?"

Being strong enough to handle the needs of dying residents hasn't hardened Marlene to bittersweet endings. She tells of a older lady who moved into the nursing home because she became so weak and confused, couldn't live alone—a familiar story.

"People come through here so fast now, it's not like the old days when you had them for a while, at least time to get to know them," Marlene recalled.

Short-term admissions of terminal patients do seem to be more and more common as hospitals can no longer afford to keep patients for lengthy stays.

"This little lady hadn't been with us a week, and she died. Turns out there was no one left for her—not a soul." Marlene needed no time to think about what she wanted to do. "She had talked once about how much she used to like getting a new dress, that it made her feel pretty," Marlene said. "So I went out and got her a new dress to be buried in. That's just something I would want done for me, that's all."

TODAY: *Comfort as you would want to be comforted.*

Born into a wealthy Russian family, Catherine De Hueck Doherty's fairy-tale life was shattered when, at 15, she entered an arranged marriage with an abusive nobleman. Catherine became a Red Cross nurses' aide at 18 and followed her husband to the World War I front, where he was a Major in the First Russian Army. "In World War I, I dipped into a sea of pain," she wrote. In 1917, during the Bolshevik Revolution, she was arrested because she was a member of the aristocracy, and was condemned to death by starvation.

These few words of introduction to Catherine Doherty reveals hers was a full, yet painful, life. Escaping to Canada from the Russian death camp Catherine devoted herself to ending poverty and racial discrimination.

Perhaps her greatest achievement was opening Listening Houses, spiritual refuges in urban environments. In 1976, at the opening of the first Listening House in Portland, Oregon, she wrote:

> People today are lonely beyond any loneliness that has embittered mankind in years past!...Perhaps it is due to our technological society. Perhaps it is due to our concern with self. Or to put it more plainly, our 'selfishness.'...The government has taken over welfare. It has taken over hospitals. It has taken over, in a word, what we used to call 'the corporal works of mercy,' but it has not noticed the terrible loneliness of man nor his alienation...Factually, a Listening House doesn't do anything, and yet it does very much.

As a caregiver you are well aware of this "terrible loneliness and alienation." And perhaps even more aware of the comforting power of simply listening.

TODAY: *Comfort by listening.*

(Reprinted with permission from *They Called Her the Baroness* by Lorene Hanley Duquin. Edmund C. Lane, S.S.P. Alba House, 2187 Victory Blvd., Staten Island, NY 10314-6603.)

Throughout history people have withdrawn from the clamor of society into monastic life, living in an abbey, monastery or convent. Part of this life is the ancient daily practice called the Consciousness Examen. Since 1548, when the Spiritual Exercises of St. Ignatius of Loyola were first published, they have served as a helpful tool for discerning one's heart and mind.

The Examen (named that because it helps us examine our lives) involves five steps:
• Enlighten
• Reflect
• Review
• Regret
• Resolve

First we look inward and ask for a fresh insight or awareness derived from our day. What did I see in myself today? What new understanding did I gain about life? It can be as simple as, "I noticed how much I enjoy tucking my residents in at night."

Second, we reflect on this "a ha!" moment. What does it mean? What can I do with this information?

Third, we review or survey our day's actions. Did I benefit others today?

At the fourth step we pause to notice any sadness or sorrow we feel about our actions today. We're not beating ourselves up, just noting what we regret and pledging to move forward.

Lastly, in step five we resolve to incorporate this new awareness or enlightenment into our way of life.

The Examen is not an exercise we do a set number of times and then graduate. Rather, this quiet self-questioning is a practice to which we can turn throughout our lives. As long as we seek answers and a sense of purpose and meaning, we can use the Examen to turn inward.

TODAY: *Comfort yourself with the Examen.*

Dr. Elisabeth Kubler-Ross, a psychiatrist, published her first book, *On Death and Dying*, in 1969, and changed the way the world regards the subject. A citizen of the U.S. and Switzerland, she has published nine books dealing with the natural phenomenon of dying.

The medical community didn't discuss death until Dr. Kubler-Ross brought it out of the dark. No research was conducted or best practices shared about this taboo subject. Of course, earlier cultures and civilizations, particularly the aboriginal and native peoples, had rituals for handling every aspect of death. Family and friends were clear about their roles, while the dying person was free from fear or isolation.

Kubler-Ross wrote:

> The most beautiful people we have known are those who have known defeat, known suffering, known struggle, known loss, and have found their way out of the depths. These people have an appreciation, sensitivity, and an understanding of life that fills them with compassion, gentleness, and deep loving concern. Beautiful people do not just happen.

Look around you. Look in the mirror. Beautiful people do not just happen. On those days when the suffering is intense, remember what happens when you live in a hot-house. You bloom.

TODAY: *Comfort and grow.*

When I am an old lady, I will still find great pleasure in talking about my friend Lynne Rosedahl, a professional certified nursing assistant. Lynne's approach to her work is so far beyond the job description, she takes my breath away. Maybe it is that soft Tennessee accent—I'm not sure—I just feel Lynne is singing a lullaby when she speaks.

One morning Lynne arrived at work to learn her favorite resident was crying uncontrollably. No one could calm the frantic woman, and there was a general consensus it may be time to give her a sedative. Maybe they should just call the doctor.

Lynne quickly learned that tears were caused by tragic news: the poor woman's healthy husband, who lived in their home, had died of a massive heart attack. She was a now a widow.

"There was only one thing I could do. I just crawled up in bed with her and I rocked her until she couldn't cry anymore."

TODAY: *Comfort like a mother.*

A nurse at St. Patrick's Residence in Naperville, Illinois, wrote this recollection:

> I was finishing my calls when a CNA stopped me in the hall and told me I should go to 2 West. She gave me the room number and resident's name. She said that the resident didn't look good to her.
>
> We sang and prayed and I anointed her. The aide left with a big smile. Just one hour later, the Lord called this resident home—a surprise to some, but not to me. Because of the caring presence of this CNA, who was a friend, I was able to comfort the family by relating the visit we had with their mom. All because of a CNA who cared.

Call it instinct or a sixth sense, but good caregivers become highly aware of the end times. Acutely sensitive to the smallest changes in a patient's condition, they feel compelled to report immediately to the supervisor and others. Thankfully, the nurse listened and didn't delay. Yes, there are always more phone calls to make and paperwork to fill out. Moments to provide care or comfort, however, cannot wait. Let us pay attention to those tiny tugs on our hearts that say, "Go now."

TODAY: *Comfort without delay.*

Mothers are famous for self-doubt or worse. My husband is good at announcing, "Listen to how you are beating yourself up!" Here's the routine: I hear a mother describe some amazing experience she had with her child, or a child sing her mom's praises, and I fret: "I never had time to do that; I was always working."

An especially sore spot is that I didn't provide Elliot any siblings until he hit age 10, when my marriage to Thurmond brought Chelsea, then 14, into the family. For years Elliot had longed for a brother or sister, but I remained single. And I've always felt terrible that I failed him.

Another divorced mother tortures herself for raising two sons without a father. Though her boys are now grown and successful men, JoAnn continues to see herself as having let the boys down.

Recently I read of a study that shows a strong correlation between the early loss of a parent and genius. Joseph Conrad, Isaac Newton, Beethoven and Virginia Woolf all lost parents at an early age. The study found that fully one-third of geniuses lost one parent by age 10, a much higher percentage than normal. JoAnn will be speechless! And I'm sure if I root around enough on the Internet, I could find a study that suggests only children are smarter or cuter or funnier or something.

Is your life half-empty or half-full? Are you a victim or a survivor? Regardless of our life experience, why not look for the benefits and see the best? Odds are, there's a study out there that suggests you're gifted!

TODAY: *Comfort yourself and see your best.*

Though she had worked at the Ohio nursing home for 16 years, most people only knew Myrna as the Menu Lady. When a new resident is admitted to the facility, Myrna sits down and learn likes and dislikes.

"I'm the one who discovers their preferences. I make sure they don't receive any foods they hate, and I make especially sure they get their favorites at least once a week," Myrna said, forgetting her shyness for a moment. A petite and quiet woman, Myrna had been coaxed to talk about her work. She clearly regarded her intake interview with new folks as a vital assignment.

But today, Myrna was talking about her early connection with residents to make another point.

"People seem to forget that I know everyone who lives here. After all, I am one of the first employees residents meet when they move in."

"So when someone dies, I would like to be told. You know how I find out now? I get a note that says, 'Don't make up a tray anymore for Mrs. So-and-So.' That hurts. I knew them, too."

By expressing herself at a staff meeting, Myrna sensitized coworkers to her situation, reminding everyone that all departments truly serve and care for the residents. Out of respect for the life that has ended, as well as the relationship all staff have with the deceased, the facility developed a communication protocol for informing everyone of a resident death.

TODAY: *Comfort all staff.*

Gathered around the large table, friends and family members of residents talked about what they would like to see done differently at the nursing facility.

"We do our best to make this institution feel like home, but we know we can do better. What would you like to see?" asked the social services director.

Nancy had come to the meeting to advocate for her friend, Elise who, at age 93, had recently moved in.

"Elise has no relatives. She is the last of her family. She has had so many losses. I wish you could help her deal with the losses."

Government regulations frame virtually every action that occurs in a nursing home, from meals to the number of dresser drawers per person. Rules about dealing with loss are murkier. What can be done when the rug is pulled out from under someone's life?

Losing one's health, independence, home, privacy and savings would make the strongest individual shaky. Where there are no family members to buffer the loss, more is required of professional caregivers.

Listen. Acknowledge. Avoid minimizing the loss, or putting on a bubbly affect. You can't possibly imagine the pain, so don't diminish it. At the same time, introduce a few new thoughts into every conversation. Has Elise met Mildred Dorne yet? They both graduated from Swarthmore. Would she be interested in a pen pal from your list of foster children? Would she consider writing some of her childhood memories to share with the Girl Scouts when they visit next week?

TODAY: *Comfort both endings and beginnings.*

As a child who loved sugar, I found Valentine's Day to be a grand occasion. Two days after my own birthday, the holiday left me on a frosting high the whole week! Our mothers made pink cupcakes and cookies to accompany the red punch and candy hearts. The last hour of the school day, we had our party.

All subject areas were involved in valentine preparations. In art class, we created elaborately-decorated boxes for receiving individual valentines from other students. The rule was always the same: "If you give any valentines, you must give them to everyone." Most teachers policed this portion of the party, counting envelopes to make sure we had enough for everyone before we were allowed to distribute.

But in this imperfect world, everyone didn't always get a card from everyone else. I looked through mine a hundred times one year, searching for something from Greg Ludlow. I remember crying to my mother about this slight, looking for comfort.

Perhaps these vivid memories are one reason I was so touched by Liz's comments about the Union House Valentine Party. Adorable handmade paper pouches, covered with pink and silver glitter, hung from each resident's door. The week before the holiday, Liz, who works in activities at my local facility, sat down with a group of residents to cut and color and paste old-fashioned valentines. "We make sure everyone gets a valentine," she said. A simple enough statement, but what a noble goal! Recalling my broken heart when Greg declared no love, I thanked Liz for caring.

TODAY: *Comfort with love.*

Strong religious faith helps speed recovery from depression among older individuals.

"Older persons with an intrinsically motivated religious faith may indeed be more able to cope with changes in their physical health and living circumstances," according to researchers at Duke University Medical Center in Durham, North Carolina.

For just under a year, the researchers used diagnostic interviews to track the emotional well-being of 94 individuals, each of whom was over 60 years of age and had been diagnosed as suffering from depression upon discharge from the hospital after illness or injury.

Some of their tests and questions focused on the study participant's own level of inner religiosity. To ascertain this level of inner faith, researchers used a 10-question assessment test that had been developed with the help of Christian ministers and Jewish rabbis.

The Duke team says that during the course of their study more than half (54 percent) of the participants recovered from their depression.

Religion seemed to help in that recovery. "Depressed patients with higher intrinsic (inner) religiosity scores had more rapid remissions than patients with lower scores," according to the study. In fact, the researchers found that patients recovered from depression 70% sooner with every 10-point increase in the religiosity assessment test score.

They speculate that, "religious faith may provide such persons with a sense of hope that things will turn out all right regardless of their problems and, thus, foster greater motivation to achieve emotional recovery."

They urged caregivers to initiate inquiries into a patient's religious faith, especially when patients are depressed, since "these beliefs may bring comfort and facilitate coping."

TODAY: *Comfort by asking about faith.*

Government inspection of healthcare facilities is often criticized for taking a snapshot in time, a report on one day, as opposed to a more complete picture of the home.

Arguments can be made for and against the value of such a snapshot.

Working in a residential setting with frail and vulnerable elders, your days are full of snapshots. Your career is a virtual photo album of high and low moments.

Jo Hogan, a career certified nursing assistant working for Beverly Healthcare at Sleepy Hollow Manor in Annandale, Virginia, says not all such snapshots are 'Kodak moments'. The Queen of the Eastern Shore Leadership Council, an honor bestowed for her 30 years of service, Jo tells a story.

"We had taken care of this woman for several years, and she had never had a visitor. The day two grown children showed up we were shocked. I didn't know she had any family."

Their mother was dying, and through some miracle, the nursing home social worker had convinced them to visit.

"Right in front of her, and she was still conscious, they fought about who would get her few remaining possessions." Other Council members listening to Jo's story nodded, having witnessed similar family battles.

"But that wasn't the worst of it. As they got ready to leave, again in front of their mother, they said to me, 'We don't have time to handle the funeral, so you take care of it, okay?' Of course I said 'yes,'" Jo says.

True to her word, Jo and her co-workers worked with the funeral home, got a dress for their resident to be buried in and, finally, attended the funeral.

We will never know what damage occurred in this family for a mother to be so poorly treated. And it is not our job to judge the children's actions. Our job in such situations is to imitate the actions of Queen Jo.

TODAY: *Comfort without judging.*

Death is the event none of us can deny or avoid forever—even the procrastinators among us. Sooner or later, we will all breathe our last breath.

A chorus of regrets often accompanies death's inevitable appearance. If the dying individual has some warning, s/he may spend her or his last days reviewing old hurts and disappointments, asking "what if" and "why me?"

Central figures in the life of the terminally ill also can experience reflection and regret. Suddenly, the time they were going to "get around to it" is no longer. Reconciliation, forgiveness or simply saying, "I love you" are not possible.

Vanessa, an LPN for more than 20 years in Indiana, had been taking care of a quiet little lady a short while. "I am always singing," Vanessa says, "usually hymns. One day, this lady asked me what I was humming, and I told her it was a hymn we sang at my church. She seemed very interested and asked me more about it. She asked me if I would take her to my church."

"I told her that, God willing, I would do just that. The next day when I came to work, I learned she had died the night before. I always have felt badly that I didn't get her to my church," Vanessa said.

Thinking logically, Vanessa couldn't possibly fault herself for not getting her resident to church. But regrets are rarely logical. Like Vanessa, we wish we could do something over again, or be given an extra hour with someone. We can't. What we can do is pledge to listen respectfully to others, because more than anything, people want to be heard. And, when feasible, grant final wishes.

TODAY: *Comfort by listening to final wishes.*

I remember reading the results of a study conducted by a healthcare chaplain on the importance of the chaplain in the lives of nursing home residents. The study interviewed both chaplains and residents, asking them essentially the same questions.

I remember little else about the study, other than the amusing conclusion. While the views held by both parties seemed to track pretty closely, the results regarding the importance of the chaplain to the residents' well-being were dramatically different. The study showed chaplains thought they were more important than residents perceived.

My friend Rev. Regis Cummings, a nursing home chaplain for more than 20 years, tells a story about how caregivers share in his work. New on the job, Regis was looking for profound experiences with nursing home patients, believing he had much to offer spiritually to older parishioners.

"I had comforted a female resident over the death of her sister," Regis said. "It was a particularly sad occasion, because she had learned of her sister's death reading the obituaries." Regis stayed with the grieving woman and offered prayer and consolation. A few days later, he returned to the facility to check on her.

Walking into the woman's room, Regis asked how she was adjusting to the news of her sister's passing. "Who are you?" the bewildered resident asked.

"I had been secretly congratulating myself for serving her so well," Regis admitted. This wake-up call brought Regis back to earth, and was the beginning of an important awareness. "That same day, I watched a nursing assistant finish helping a resident get in bed by tucking a little teddy bear under her arm. I saw that simple gesture provided much more comfort than I probably ever could. I saw the greatness of the nursing assistant."

TODAY: *Comfort in little ways.*

My mother is one of them. So is an old family friend. I am referring to people who decide that the death of their beloved pet was so painful they will never own another dog.

Over the past 15 years, I have met a few caregivers who have told me that death has driven them out of the profession. In the majority of cases, I hear they "needed a break" from seeing patients they love die: "I took a few years off and worked in a store. When I was ready, I came back, because I missed the people."

Knowing our own limitations and needs is critically important to maintaining good physical and emotional health. I remember Melissa, a nurses' aide in Tennessee, telling me she had to get a change of scenery. No one could talk Melissa out of what they perceived as a crazy move: a factory job. She refused a change of assignment and even a leave of absence. Melissa knew what she needed and she took care of herself. A few months later, a refreshed and renewed Melissa was back at work, more lighthearted than ever.

Melissa didn't run away; she consciously created her own plan of care. There is no way Melissa can stop loving others. She will always be affected by the death of her dear residents.

When we declare an experience so painful we cannot risk another, it is important to recognize what is actually happening. My mom loves life, and whether it is a dog or a human being, she will always grieve the passing of life. She can't stop loving, and we're glad!

Feeling sorrow and grief is a powerful reminder of our humanity. Yes, it is hard, but it is also precious. Life is like that.

TODAY: *Comfort yourself with time-outs.*

We all enjoy stories of love at first sight. Across a crowded room, they instantly know, and strangers become lovers.

Such near-mystical tales give life its gilt edge, providing the golden glow we all long to believe in. Surely there is more to this world than earning money to buy things and pay bills?

Millie Aldrich's story of receiving a message from the dead bears this same shimmering quality, reminding us again that there is so much about life we will never fully understand.

A nurse aide for more than two decades, Millie gets attached to her residents, and the attachment is mutual. Just over five feet tall with a ready smile, Millie truly loves to serve others, and specializes in the smallest of comforts. She is called the Ice Lady where she works in northern Indiana, but not because she is cold! Every afternoon Millie freshens the water pitchers in each resident's room, dispensing ice and cheeriness.

One of the men she cared for was clearly dying. Millie was close to her residents, and said she had always felt a strong and inexplicable bond with this gentleman. Later that day, he died.

"I was so upset, just devastated by his death," Millie says, adding that her mysterious friendship with the resident had made his death more difficult than others. While she knew she would get over it, Millie was upset.

The next day, a delivery truck appeared at Millie's home with a package. Inside, she found a music box, a final gift from the deceased older man. "You can't imagine what that did for me," Millie says.

TODAY: *Find comfort in mystery.*

Today is my Grandma Catherine Purcell's birthday. She was born in 1904, and has lived her entire life in the Boston area. For almost 10 years, she has lived in Braintree Manor.

My grandparents were my first pen pals. I loved receiving mail, and especially something from them. "Enclosed, a bookmark," Grandpa would write, directing me to the $5 bill in the envelope.

After she became a widow, my Gram moved to a smaller place, then to a nursing home. I had always memorized the Purcell addresses: 1349 William Morrissey Boulevard, 191 Fenno Street, and 80 Clay Street. When Gram moved into the nursing home, I stopped committing her address to memory. Maybe if I couldn't remember the zip code in Braintree, she would eventually go home.

But she has stayed there, as one ailment after another further compromised any chances she had of moving back home. A few years ago she stopped opening her eyes, and now she can't see. I kept up the mail for a long time; my aunt would read my letters to Gram when she visited. But after a while, I felt odd sending letters to someone who never answered and sometimes wasn't sure who I was. Birthdays and Christmas became especially tough, as I couldn't think of a thing Gram needed. Another nightgown? Some chocolates?

One day, in the middle of something else, I knew what I had to do. I would begin sending gifts to the staff that care for my Gram. They long ago became her primary family, the ones who see her thousands of hours more than I do every year. This year, I sent some books and angel garlands to her caregivers, thanking them for being there for her and for us.

TODAY: *Comfort the comforters.*

Being a city girl, I still pay a great deal of attention to man-made signs of seasonal changes. Watching for annual cycles, my country-born husband is more tuned in to trees and plants.

I get a great kick out of a nearby farmer who puts his bird-feeders and Christmas wreath out on Thanksgiving Day and takes them down on Easter. I have my own personal signs of the seasons, such as the transfer in late September of summer clothes from my bedroom to the guest room clos-et and then back again, joyously, in May.

I remember when, every April, my mom tried in vain to con-vince my brother, Will, the cotton short-sleeved shirts she pulled from a large steamer trunk were his. "No!" he stomped, refusing to give up his long-sleeved flannel shirts. We have more than one family summer vacation picture of Will sweltering in flannel.

Healthcare institutions work hard to create visual cues and rituals for residents and patients, signaling changes in the weather, date and coming holidays. But how well do we inform one another that a death has occurred in our extend-ed family?

Death can be an awkward event to announce, particularly to those who are fast reaching the same passage. Simple, rev-erent rituals can greatly reduce the tension and sorrow that surrounds death.

As Andre Dubus so eloquently phrases it, "For ritual allows those who cannot will themselves out of the secular to per-form the spiritual as dancing allows the tongue-tied man a ceremony of love."

Why not sit down with members of your facility's commu-nity at large and explore respectful gestures you could for-malize for informing one another of a death? Ask residents, their families, staff and volunteers what they would like to do to acknowledge someone's passing. Create death rituals.

TODAY: *Comfort with rituals.*

Amanda was a nurse in CNA clothing. A single mother of two, she didn't have the time or money to go to nursing school, though she certainly had the brains and instincts.

Amanda was highly regarded by her coworkers. Though she had worked for less than a year at the Alabama facility, Amanda knew the protocols and staff and stayed well-informed on resident admissions and discharges. She also wrote poetry, finding such self-expression a good way to deal with some of the daily stresses of work.

When the senior aide position was posted, Amanda knew it was hers. "Some of the girls even came up to me and said, 'Amanda, you have to apply for that job, its you!' and I was embarrassed, but I agreed. It was perfect for me."

Amanda didn't get the job. To everyone's amazement, management filled the job solely based on seniority, which meant Amanda didn't even get an interview.

She quit. Furious with the decision, which she perceived as wrong for the residents as well as for her, Amanda walked out and never came back. Today, she is in nursing school, motivated in part by her pain.

Institutional life is full of compromises, oversights, and yes, imperfect decisions. Life itself is not always fair. When you see someone caught in the crossfire of inequity and injustice, give them comfort. You may not be able to change the circumstances, but you can take away some of their pain.

TODAY: *Comfort those in pain.*

We don't talk easily about our money.

Early in life, we learn wages and earnings are private matters, and we are socialized to not ask others about their pay. Perhaps this "no trespassing" attitude is part of the reason we freak out when we learn what other people are paid.

Does anything get people more incensed at work than finding out someone else earns more than they do?

Here's the story: Ann had 23 years of working in dietary behind her. The last nine she had been the department head. Courted by a new facility, Ann was offered the directorship of a gleaming kitchen plus a 25-percent increase in salary. Conflicted out of loyalty to her current employer, Ann went to him to discuss her dilemma.

Brad didn't want to lose Ann. She was a terrific employee, known to stay under budget. She was also well-liked by her staff, and a creative chef. However, Brad was honest. "I can't offer you any new kitchen equipment, unless we replace the walk-in cooler later in the year. I could come pretty close on the raise, though."

Ann decided to stay, and somehow word of the raise leaked out. A self-taught cook, Ann had no formal education beyond high school. The other department heads, several with master's degrees, were enraged! How dare the administrator be strong-armed by Ann? Blinded by their sense of unfairness, Ann's co-workers began to distance themselves from her, gossiping about whether she even had a real job offer.

One by one, the aggrieved department chiefs paraded into Brad's office, making their individual cases for a raise. Based on merit and performance, several associates were certain they deserved a pay increase equal to or greater than Ann's.

For whatever his reasons, Brad gave no other raises. Consequently, two department heads were actively job-hunting, one was getting madder by the minute, and the others were expressing various levels of discontent.

Just as promotions based strictly on seniority seem unfair, raises given outside the normal process are equally maddening. Yesterday's words seem worth repeating: When you see someone caught in the crossfire of inequity and injustice, give them comfort. You may not be able to change any of the circumstances, but you can take away some of their pain.

TODAY: *Comfort the aggrieved.*

Teamwork and consensus management are terms progressive administrators use to describe their style of running a healthcare residence. In assisted living facilities, the universal worker is a popular staffing model, permitting one individual to work in a variety of settings...efficient for the employer and interesting for the employee.

Talking about the value of teamwork is a lot easier than actually working as a team. Teams are not hierarchical. Rather, they are based on principles of equality and shared responsibility. No one player is more important on a high-functioning team.

Most of the nursing staff at a California facility had reached the same conclusion: the bath schedule was not working. More and more residents preferred baths at night. The day shift was falling behind on bathing, due to heavier-care patients requiring more time for feeding, therapies and rest. All factors seemed to lead to one solution: accommodate resident and staff wishes by giving a good percentage of baths at night.

Having talked informally for weeks, a group of nurses and CNAs wrote a simple proposal to the Director of Nursing. From start to finish, they described how the change in bathing could work, and the expected benefits. With excitement, the team submitted their proposal to the director of nursing services....who promptly rejected it with no reason given. When pressed by nurses, the DNS simply replied, "Because I said so." Case closed.

Morale has hit bottom, and anger is rising. Rather than working with her concerned staff, she shut down communication. Unfortunately, this scenario is not too uncommon. Top nursing home management still believe in veto power and, worse yet, they use it.

TODAY: *Comfort the disappointed.*

Lucy delivers afternoon snacks in her facility. A cheery flight attendant coming down the aisle, Lucy looks forward to her duties like a party planner.

"It's my chance to spread a little good will," she chirps. Lucy is a social bug, and has always been the one to remember people's birthdays and anniversaries, to show up at wakes and funerals. Some of her coworkers tease, "You're the social director of the Love Boat!"

The smiling faces of residents keep Lucy going. "I always try and get them to laugh or smile before I leave the room. If I don't, I just don't feel right."

At her age, Lucy should know that not everyone can be plumped up like a pillow into a good mood. Some folks are just plain sour, and no amount of sweetness changes the balance.

Barbara is just such a patient, a life-long complainer. Having lived most of her life in mental hospitals, Barbara is well acquainted with how to file grievances and stir up the hornets. Unless she is recalling a particularly successful time she got on someone's case, Barbara is dour and nasty. To Lucy, she is that elusive challenge, that ragged nail that needs to be filed.

"I can't stand it!" Lucy said late one afternoon, "No matter what I do, Barbara is so snotty to me! I know she just hates me."

Try as we might, none of us can control the feelings or behavior of others. Each of us is governed by our own temperament and will. If, despite Lucy's friendliest attempts, Barbara stays stuck in the mud, that is a reflection on Barbara, not on Lucy. The old schoolyard wisdom, "don't take it personally," applies here.

TODAY: *Comfort the discontent.*

Most caregivers have their little rules, some of them close to superstitions, about patterns that occur in institutions. "Deaths come in waves," we tell one another, remembering how no one died in October and then in November five residents passed away.

Whether there is any rationale for when bad or sad things happen, we agree the cumulative effects of grief can be unbearable. Sometimes we wonder if we will find the grace and strength to move on.

Such was the case at Verdelle Village when Sherrie, a beloved nurses' aide, died in a car accident on her way to work. Sherrie was the strong one everyone relied upon. For years she had provided high-quality care in this northern Vermont facility.

What made Sherrie's death even more painful was that a coworker was the first one to come upon the accident. We all know in this work coworkers can become as close as family. Sherrie's injuries were massive; the medical examiner declared she had died instantly. The prolonged suffering occurred a few miles down the road, at the facility. Staff and residents were hit hard by Sherrie's tragic and violent death.

The idea of a memorial service for Sherrie conducted in the facility gained momentum. Everyone needed a focus for their energy, a way of paying tribute to their fallen coworker. Days later, a program with music and eulogies was held in the facility multipurpose room. Staff and residents attended and tears were shed. Sherrie received the loving good-bye she deserved, and healing began.

TODAY: *Comfort one another.*

Mourners are susceptible to illness—more susceptible because they are grieving.

The effects of behavioral factors on immune measurements have been proven by a variety of studies. Looking at negative states and traits, researchers have found definite links between bereavement, depression and divorce and low immunity and poor resistance to illness. Chronic stress and pessimism increase blood levels of Epstein-Barr virus, associated with chronic fatigue syndrome.

What does this tell us?

During times of loss and negative energy, human beings need a dose of positivity to stay healthy. Personal sharing and support, humor, exercise and relaxation will increase white blood cells and endorphins.

Knowing about these connections, we can enhance the well-being of others and ourselves when tough times hit. Comforting someone who is going through a divorce or dealing with a death is not easy. Avoid pressuring yourself to find just the right thing to say. Offering condolences and sympathy is an art few of us practice regularly. Suggesting you take a walk together, enjoy a massage or take in a fun movie can be just what the doctor would order.

TODAY: *Comfort creatively.*

Diana L. Whaley, a CNA in Tarboro, NC., has comforted thousands of frightened patients during more than two decades of caring. Named Certified Nursing Assistant of the Year by the North Carolina Health Care Association in 1999, Diana pays attention to details as well as to the big picture. Listening to the fears expressed by many of her patients and their families, Diana realized the need to set the record straight.

Horror stories aired on television had made new residents dread moving into a nursing home. She saw a need to reassure the public, to tell them there was nothing to fear. Diana wrote a letter to local newspapers and television stations stressing that the great majority of nursing homes are wonderful, loving places for North Carolinians in need.

> People enter a nursing home because they need round-the-clock care—care the family may not be able to provide because both spouses work or because family members are either scattered and distant, very few, or nonexistent. Most people do not prepare for long-term health care. They do not want to think of losing their independence, their inability to do the simple activities of daily living such as bathing, dressing, feeding themselves, ambulation and toileting. No one wants to think of death or dying. Those are the real fears—not fear of neglect and abuse.

> The media and lawyers capitalize on the frustrations of the residents and of the family members. Another contributing factor is society's attitude toward caregivers. We must raise public consciousness about the true role of the caregivers. It is not a burden to work with old, frail and sometimes dying people; it's a privilege. There is not a more noble profession to belong to. The nursing home CNA provides quality and special care to our society's elders.

> As a caregiver, I am tired of hearing and reading of only the problems and mistakes associated with nursing homes. Too much attention is given to failures, and the

conduct of those few reflects unfairly on the many who serve with a sense of pride, commitment, and professionalism. We must support and encourage the reputable facilities and operators. We need to raise public awareness of the positive contributions CNAs make to the health and well-being of the nursing facility residents.

TODAY: *Comfort with truth.*

March: Blessed are the meek, for they shall inherit the earth.

To be meek is not to be weak. Meekness means we don't spit when we give our opinion, but our opinion is still given. Gentle souls aren't proud, obnoxious or pushy and they aren't doormats, either. You are surrounded by the meek; they work behind the scenes, quietly seeing what needs to be done and getting it done.

For many of us, force is a more attractive way of doing right. We fight the war on drugs and the war on poverty, believing force must be met with force. In truth, force is endlessly met with force. Impatient and even angry for change, we come out swinging, oblivious to the casualties of our private wars.

Aggression flows through generations, as we rear our children to carry our cries and causes. In the Holy Land and Northern Ireland, land was seized centuries ago by people who believed resistance would end when witnesses died. But memories don't die; they are passed on to youth who feel destined to restore their people's honor.

Our only hope, in our homes, workplaces and world is for the meek to inherit, to take over, and to lead us into a peaceful day where respect for one another is paramount. Neither harsh nor aggressive, meek human beings are self-controlled, knowing they can get much farther making their point without poking anyone in the eye. Hard to rile or irritate, gentle caregivers will more likely laugh off the annoying, seeing charm rather than harm.

Meek leaders are submissive authorities; they understand that gentleness only enhances their strength and influence. Meek followers are also submissive, submissive to their inner sense of love and duty, free from force.

father died in a nursing home from decubitus ulcers (pressure sores). It was horrible. My lifetime goal is to make decubitus ulcers a household word so that my father will not have died in vain. Decubitus ulcers is a very real problem because there isn't enough staff in any capacity to turn the bedridden every two hours.

I am so rewarded visiting nursing homes. Residents cry with happiness when hugged. A basic need of humanity is not being met. One resident was in a state-of-the-art room and she might as well have been on a deserted island. Her son lived 30 minutes away and was "too busy" to visit. Research shows babies die from lack of touch and monkeys would rather be physically loved than fed.

As a nation we should adopt the term "Grandpeople" rather than elders. It's a new day in the nursing home and we need new terms. Together we can change things. We have a Humane Society segment on the local news, where dogs and cats are shown for adoption. Adopt-a-highway is all over the nation. I want pictures and stories about nursing home residents broadcast as an adopt-a-grandperson news segment. Even if they have a family, families can adopt someone and visit, making sure basic needs are met. Visits could be daily or weekly. Involving the adopters' extended family would multiply the help in nursing homes overnight.

I think once people realize that grandpeople are sponges for love they will join a huge volunteer effort, making it easier for nurses and CNAs to do their jobs. My quest is to give respect, honor and love to our grandpeople.

—Sherry Ernst
www.nodecubitus.com

TODAY: *Be in creation, not reaction.*

What is it with big talkers? Just because we are the only creatures with the gift of speech, do we think we're supposed to use it all the time?

If that's the case, we've got double the number of ears and eyes, so doesn't that mean we should be spending a lot more time observing and listening? Do the math: just 20 percent of the time should be allotted for talking.

My dreams are a source of great personal amusement. While others may shake their heads when I tell my latest nighttime tale, I am totally entertained. A few nights ago I dreamt about a brand-new, incredibly cheap long-distance phone service. I couldn't believe it, one cent a minute! One! My dreamself e-mailed my son, and he was the voice of reason: "Mom, there is no way. Read the fine print; there is some hook, some fee or service charge. Check it out; I just can't believe one cent a minute."

Working hard in my dream world, I did plenty of research, read all about the new service on the Internet, and even questioned the telemarketer. No hidden charges. A flat one cent a minute, 24 hours a day, 365 days a year, anywhere in the U.S.. So I signed up.

My first phone call was to my doubting son. Only then did I learn the phone service was cheap because I couldn't talk and be heard—I could only listen. Hmmm...what a concept!

Listening is a powerful source of goodwill, strength, energy and happiness. Listening can answer your greatest questions. Listen to what people say about you in your presence. What conclusions have they drawn about you? How are you perceived?

Don't listen as an insecure soul, needing to be built up and praised by the outside world. Just listen to discover if what you know about yourself is actually showing up. You know yourself as a caregiver with high personal and professional standards. Is that how you're received?

TODAY: *Listen for confirmations.*

Angels Among Us

There are angels among us
Without any wings,
But they fly just the same,
Doing many kinds of things.
The fly up and down halls
On feet that may ache.
But they keep on smiling
With backs ready to break.
They cook our meals and serve them.
They help us bathe and dress.
They make our beds and clean our rooms
But are they angels? Yes!
There are angels among us
Who give us our pills.
And pass out the medicine
To help ease our ills.
Some angels entertain us
And help to make us laugh.
Though you may call them aides or nurses,
Housekeepers, cooks or staff.
Here's something we want to tell you
That I feel we don't say enough.
Thanks for all the things you do!
You're each one an angel to us!

—Anna Jean Allen, daughter of Era Watson,
resident of Winston County Nursing Home, Louisville, MS

TODAY: *See the angels.*

Being bilingual today isn't limited to speaking a foreign language. Bilingual individuals are those who can communicate between two or more different worlds.

My mother is taking a computer class for beginners. No doubt the instructor knows computers well; she just can't speak the language of the computer-illiterate. What is needed is someone who can talk with folks in everyday terms and introduce the high-tech world at the same time.

More and more employers are seeking such bilingual individuals. Law firms are hiring mediators. Financial planning offices are adding social workers to help clients deal with the emotional issues around retirement, feuding families and money itself.

The best caregivers are cross-talkers, comfortable with the residents and families, as well as with supervisors and new hires. I remember my first few weeks working as a nursing assistant. Mrs. Martin has CA. Arnold in room 107 has COPD. What??

Answering complicated questions with gentle simplicity and responding to mean remarks with lightness, the meek caregiver manages her environment without fanfare. She respectfully says what needs to be said with a smile, and moves on.

TODAY: *Speak several languages.*

A note from a St. Patrick's Residence nurse in Naperville, Illinois:

> One of the third floor residents had a rather bad emesis (vomiting) during the noon meal. Immediately, two CNAs started the seemingly hopeless task of cleaning up. Both CNAs gave careful consideration to the dignity of the resident, going about their work without embarrassing him. They escorted him from the dining room so they could remove the soiled clothing and bathe him. During the process they reassured him, telling him all was well and that he was OK. I can remember feeling such admiration for the compassion they displayed. I wondered how many people realize that we have 'modern-day saints' working in our midst. It is an honor and a privilege to be in their daily presence.

Performing such intimate tasks requires us to be grounded in deep humility...there but by the grace of God go I. Our awkward feelings cannot be permitted to surface, for this moment is not about us. The secret of the meek is to be so present to the Other, so conscious of their needs and concerns that nothing else exists. Thoughts about self are suspended and energy is concentrated on pure service, freeing both parties of tension.

Without question, I am certain the gentleman who was helped by these two gracious aides now regards them with tremendous affection, if not love. When we reach out with such compassion, we do indeed inherit the earth.

TODAY: *Concentrate on service, not on self.*

If you want something done, ask a busy person. That's the street talk, right?

In my lifetime, and particularly in my small town, it's true. I look at who serves on the school board, volunteer ambulance squad, and charity events and the same trusted names appear. Why is that? Are these folks just better people than the rest of us, or more organized, or hyperactive? Are they independently wealthy? Maybe they're just well-disciplined?

I don't happen to believe any of those factors make busy people more productive. What makes them stand out is their decision to serve. While the rest of us talk about not being able to find the time, they make the time. Like being in love, deciding to serve is not a feeling; it is an act of our will.

We get sucked in by a two-hour made-for-TV movie; they watch television only on weekends. We chat an hour on the phone that could have been spent selling popcorn at the high school basketball game, where we still could have talked with friends.

The prolific and successful artist Pablo Picasso addressed this sense of purpose in a letter to his mistress:

> Everybody has the same energy potential. The average person wastes his in a dozen little ways. I bring mine to bear in one thing only: my painting, and everything is sacrificed to it, you and everyone else, myself included.

The irony of course, is that such sacrifice is ultimately what buys one a great sense of satisfaction and peace of mind. Good caregivers know this because it is their way of life.

TODAY: *Decide to serve.*

Patient Trust

Above all, trust in the slow work of God
We are quite naturally impatient in everything
To reach the end without delay.
We should like to skip the intermediate stages.
We are impatient of being on the way to something unknown,
something new.
And yet it is the law of all progress
that it is made by passing through
some stages of instability—
and that it may take a very long time.
And so I think it is with you.
Your ideas mature gradually, let them grow,
Let them shape themselves, without undue haste.
Don't try to force them on,
As they you could be today what time
(that is to say, grace and circumstances
acting on your own good will)
will make of your tomorrow.
Only God could say what this new spirit
Gradually forming within you will be.
Give our Lord the benefit of believing
That his hand is leading you,
And accept the anxiety of feeling yourself
In suspense and incomplete.

—Pierre Teilhard de Chardin

TODAY: *Trust and be patient.*

When my husband and I first married, I was a stranger in his musician world. A cellist, he played with the Vermont Philharmonic Orchestra and a chamber group. He was either practicing, rehearsing or performing, terms I misused for months.

I often would tell someone Thurmond was practicing when he was actually rehearsing.

He would say with the patience of a new lover:

> Honey, when I practice, I am working on different pieces of music as well as my technique, my bowing, fingering, the basics. I practice by myself, getting to the point where I will be able to play the pieces with others. When I rehearse, I am with the other members of the orchestra or chamber group, and we are playing together until we are good enough to perform for a live audience.

The distinction of practicing is important to understand when considering any discipline, not just music. One's practice is what she does routinely, the fundamentals of a larger picture. We refer to the practice of law, the practice of medicine, of opening up an accounting practice.

What is your practice? What do you work on daily, striving to become more and more adept? I once sat at a fundraising dinner and watched the keynote speaker as she was introduced. The host digressed from the short biography the speaker had prepared, and was sharing some of her own impressions. The guest speaker was amazed at the incidents and examples from her life being shared. Through the eyes of another, the speaker's practice was revealed: a kind and caring soul, a purveyor of generous acts. Over time, her giving had become easier, sweeter, more frequent...a true practice.

TODAY: *Practice for your performance.*

Yesterday I met with an employee of a state prison. She has worked in correctional facilities more than 25 years, and says she is never bored. "You never know what the day will bring," Sharon said. "I can come in here with a plan for the whole day, and it gets blown right out of the water. It's always exciting. But you gotta be flexible; if you're not, you don't belong here."

I expect this is a fair statement of fact about working in any institutional setting. Yes, when we are working with a large number of people, order and routine is mandatory. But the best-laid plans are often bumped by something more pressing....like a break in the sewer line or a flu epidemic. Making plans in advance is always wise, but giving them too much weight or importance is not. I've watched grown men and women fall apart when a staffing crisis requires them to work as a floater on a different wing. You would think they were being sent to the Bering Straits to bob around on an iceberg!

Our tendency is to seek the security and predictability of a plan, thinking it takes away fear, or the unknown. Our plans merely give the mind something concrete to fix on, and can actually serve as a distraction. While we are busy trying to control a situation, we can easily miss the mysteries around us, and not notice the presence of unexpected beauty or good fortune.

Changes in duties, patients, policies and procedures are all disruptive. But change is the stuff of life. Who knows? The wing you are transferred to, the new partner you work with, could be the beginning of your happiest days. Remain open to change, and beware of the limitation of a plan. After all, it is a four-letter word.

TODAY: *Stay flexible.*

We're told there is an artist inside each one of us. I decided it was time to get acquainted with mine, so I enrolled in a class with Peter Wilkes, a master in the teaching and painting of religions icons. Our class met for a week, and we transformed blocks of wood covered with linen and rabbit skin glue into glorious replicas of ancient portraits of Jesus.

Icon paining is about watching the teacher, but it is also about listening to his coaching: "Don't work so hard, you work it too hard. Just drop and float the paint. Let the bath do its thing, get out of the way. Don't play with it. Never go back, you can't go back. Watch it, as each day it comes more to life. The icon will heal itself."

Rereading Peter's instructions, I saw how they applied perfectly to my life. I do work it too hard, and I do get in the way. Sometimes I can't be easy with anything. I go over and over a sore point until it is even sorer. I do play with it, rather than trusting that things work out for the best.

Never go back; you can't go back. How many of us long for the good old days which, upon closer reflection, weren't all that good anyway? Once I drove to my grandmother's summer home, which I hadn't seen in years. The new owner had taken our wonderful screened porch and turned it into a bar, complete with those little boy liquor dispensers that look like they are relieving themselves. Grandma would have died! I almost did.

Watch it, as each day it comes more to life...it will heal itself. Again, direction for my life. The more I live in a trusting way, staying loose and resisting the urge to judge, the more alive I feel. And yes, my own healing happens when I lighten up, forgive and forget. Whether we're painting an icon or doing our best to love one another, the secret is to trust and have a light touch.

TODAY: *Keep it light.*

Mary Kay wobbled into the dining room. It wasn't quite 5:30 AM, and few other residents were up and dressed.

A table for four sat like a stage prop next to the window; the radio played on the sill. Squared to the corners, a box of tissue and a straw were placed on the table, a vase of artificial flowers in the center. Draped over the arm of the chair was a terry-cloth bib.

Slowly, Mary Kay sat down, placing her large-print Bible on the table. She carefully aligned the book with the straw and adjusted the vase. With everything in order, Mary Kay tottered back to her room, returning with a large magnifying glass.

Again, she sat down at the table, making minute changes in the positioning of items. She spent considerable time finding a page in her Bible, holding her magnifying glass just so. After uttering about three words out loud, Mary Kay's head gently dropped down onto the soft pages, and she began to snore.

"Yup, that's Mary Kay's routine," a nursing assistant confirmed later in the day. "She wants us to get her up early, and have the table set just so. Once she gets out there, she usually sleeps another hour. I don't think she reads anymore."

How easy it would be to simply dismiss Mary Kay's wishes! Why go to all that trouble for someone who doesn't do anything at the table but sleep? She could just stay in her room and rest another hour.

Odds are Mary Kay has opened her days with scripture for many years. Each of us has our early routines, often involving coffee and prayer. To their credit, the nursing home staff recognized the importance to Mary Kay of keeping her routine. And who's to say or know what comfort it affords her?

TODAY: *Honor old routines.*

With 17,000 nursing homes in the United States, and assisted living facilities opening daily, we can forget that most older people around the world, our Grandpersons, are cared for at home by a relative.

A Families USA study found that, even in this country, one in four families cares for aging kin:

> The average family caregiver devotes 18 hours a week, although some 4.1 million caregivers provide at least 40 hours a week. And typically, they do so for more than four years.

> Women remain the caregivers nearly three-fourths of the time...because many had children later in life, they are caring simultaneously for both ends of the age spectrum.

The survey found 41 percent of caregivers for the elderly also had children under 18.

Can you feel the fatigue? Everyone wants mom's attention. Like a nurses' aide with eight or more Grandpersons asking for a drink of water, a change of clothes, to be put to bed...one can quickly become overwhelmed. Taking in one need at a time, counting on our inner reserve and keeping realistic standards are key techniques for managing the load.

Perhaps your facility could offer support to family caregivers. How about teaching a few night classes on the basics of special diets, transferring patients without injury, or bathing and dressing tips? I will never forget watching aides take residents in PJs into the bathroom, then seeing them emerge in their clothes!

CNAs have much to teach family caregivers: dear daughters, daughters-in-law, sisters, wives and mothers. With the weight of the world on their shoulders, they have also inherited the earth.

TODAY: *Teach other caregivers.*

Mentoring has become a common practice of good caregiving. Learning on the job, or apprenticing, is an honored tradition for many professions. Books can only be so helpful in instructing one on the nuts and bolts of a trade.

For 25 years or more I have longed for a mentor, a woman I could look up to and emulate. In college, I had a part-time job helping Lily Anna Sophia Nutt, a clever little Swedish widow in her late seventies. Working around her lovely home, full of antiques, I wished Lily would talk to me about life, about husbands and children. Sure we talked, but I imagined different kinds of conversations, where I would learn life's secrets and the moral to every story.

In my thirties, I yearned for Priscilla Smith to take me under her wing. The well-read and well-educated wife of a state senator, Priscilla was a community pillar. She supported a great range of good causes, and was a good mother and grandmother. Again, I found myself wanting to sit at the feet of a confident, successful woman. Priscilla was good to me and we shared plenty—just not what I had hoped.

A few years ago, I had a flash while walking in the woods. The mentor I had been seeking? The woman I wanted to learn from and strive toward? She was I. No one else could look at my life and draw conclusions and directions from it but me. I smiled at this realization, particularly when I saw how much I had wanted both Lily and Priscilla to be more generous with me. What I wanted from them was nothing they could give me. I had to discover what I needed and make sure I got it.

I have had three spiritual directors and a professional coach to date, and all of them have helped me on my journey. My best mentor, however, is Bethany. I decided to stop looking for that special woman and, instead, to become her.

TODAY: *Mentor yourself.*

One of my greatest joys is speaking to large groups of care-givers. The love and strength in the room is unbelievable! I always tell people I meet on planes that I have the best job in the U.S. "What are you, a stockbroker?" they ask.

"No," I tell them, "I do presentations and workshops with our nation's royal family, the caregivers."

At a downtown auditorium in Detroit, I had the privilege of opening a day-long gathering of the area's finest CNAs, working in both home health and nursing homes. With more than 350 people in the room, the morning had a joy-ous buzz. At one point, I asked my audience to share stories. "Tell me what you like to do, tell me what gives you satis-faction."

For just a moment, shyness swept the room, then suddenly conference attendees began to volunteer their stories. We were treated to a range of sweet scenes, one leading to another. As the room became quiet, I asked again, "Anyone else want to share what they like about their job?"

From the top left row someone yelled, "To wash their booties!" Laughter erupted. I could see the pursed lips of one of the conference organizers, a university lady. I knew she didn't think we were talking about knit baby socks.

"Bless you," I answered. How many others have literally refused to even consider a career in caregiving because of this duty, one of the most delicate parts of the daily assign-ment? And yet, who among us would want to sit all day with an unclean bottom, burning in discomfort?

After listening to a few of my comments, the aide who had brought down the house with her remark spoke up in a seri-ous voice, and told us how appreciative patients were of her excellent baths. Heads began to nod, as we listened careful-ly to her words. How wonderful that she could joke and be light-hearted! I'm sure she makes bath time comfortable and happy.

TODAY: *Keep people clean and comfortable.*

What is the difference between the purpose of your job and the meaning of your work?

> We must learn to distinguish between purpose and meaning in life. Purpose has something to do with being productive and setting goals and knowing what needs to be done and doing it. It is easy to have purpose. To write seven letters today, to wax that floor, to finish this legal brief, to make out those reports, to complete this degree, that's purpose.

> Meaning, on the other hand, depends on my asking myself who will care and who will profit and who will be touched and who will be forgotten, hurt or affected by my doing those things. Purpose determines what I will do with this part of my life. Meaning demands to know why I'm doing it and with what global results.

Sister Joan Chittister offers us a powerful framework for regarding our life and work. How many nursing assistants, when asked about their work, say, "Oh, I'm just a nurses' aide?"

In this holy work of yours, there is no such thing as "just." Without your tender and dependable attentions, just where do you think these individuals would live? Why on earth would you minimize the importance of your life or theirs?

Working hard to create a high-quality care environment, you risk limiting your focus to the task at hand, forgetting the thoughts and feelings behind your actions. No, you are not just brushing someone's hair or inserting a hearing aide. You are touching another person, and in this very act, acknowledging her worth and uniqueness. You are helping her prepare to greet the day and share with others.

Each day, you experience the seen and the unseen. The seen is your purpose, your job description. The unseen is your meaning, your job satisfaction.

TODAY: *Experience the unseen.*

Visiting someone who is sick or confined is not an easy assignment. Those of us least caught up in social conventions, usually children, seem the most natural when dropping by the nursing home. Yes, we remind them not to run, but we are basically grateful for their exuberance and curiosity.

When visiting or caring for the frail and vulnerable, we seek to connect with them. A pastoral care worker shared this with me, suggesting it is a good guideline for framing interaction with nursing home residents:

> Remember, they have special needs: For meaning, purpose and hope, to transcend circumstances, for support in dealing with loss, for support of religious behaviors and to engage in these behaviors, for personal dignity and a sense of worthiness, for unconditional love, to express anger and doubt, to feel that God is on their side, to love and serve others, to be thankful, to forgive and be forgiven and to prepare for death and dying. (Incidentally, I believe I share all these needs!)

To help someone meet his or her particular unexpressed needs, she further recommended we listen to what the other person brings up. "Work with what they mention as a basis for a healthy exchange. Listening is the key." Here is her list of issues to listen for:

1. Hopes and life goals
2. Major branching points and decisions in my life
3. Family
4. Career or major life work
5. Role of money in my life
6. Health and body image
7. Sexual identity or experiences
8. Loves and hates over my lifetime
9. Unfairness...times I was wronged or wronged others (disappointment, guilt)
10. Experiences with death and ideas about dying

TODAY: *Base conversations on special needs.*

We girls and our hair! How is it possible to have so many radically different hairstyles on one head in one lifetime?

My curly, thick Irish hair has defied hairdressers in several states. "You've got hair for three people on this head." "This is like the highest-quality shag carpet, more fiber per inch!"

With so many varied hairy heads running around the globe, I am glad my state requires 2,000 hours of training before issuing a beautician's license.

Professionals must have training in the classroom and on the job. For all of her training, Mindy put a rinse on my hair that looked like I had a goldfish on top of my head. Brassy? It was Cheezo-colored!

Only a veteran stylist was able to repair that accident, a man who'd had as much training as Mindy but a lot more experience. Good hairdressers, like good caregivers, learn something new every day. Those who make it look easy are the champions, combining an amazing sense of self-confidence with a vast knowledge base.

Remember the painting entitled "Whistler's Mother"? James Abbott McNeill Whistler painted it. Reportedly, Whistler said of his work, "It took me two hours to do the painting but 40 years to learn how to do it in two hours."

Gentle caregivers tell us the same thing. "It took me less than 5 minutes to convince Mr. Jones to eat his breakfast, but 25 years to learn how to do it in 5 minutes."

TODAY: *See the depth of your skill.*

Even when you think no one is watching, someone is.

I've seen you notice something wasn't quite right with a resident. Then you really pursue the problem with the nurse to find out the cause and the solution. I've seen you hold a resident's hand throughout a storm.

I've known you to knit something for a resident. I've heard you sing to the residents at night when they can't sleep.

I've seen you being 'punched out' trying to change a resident who insists s/he doesn't need changing.

I know that you came in on your day off to get a resident ready for her grandson's wedding.

I know that you gave a resident a bubble bath on her birthday so she'd feel special. I've seen you curl hair and do nails for residents who 'needed' some extra TLC.

I know that you've shopped for residents on your day off for things they need and aren't able to get on their own.

I know you carry candy in your pockets because some of the residents really like candy. I've seen you massage a resident's feet when your own must be killing you.

—Loving observations from the nurses of
St. Patrick's Residence, Naperville, Illinois.

TODAY: *Know you are noticed.*

Even in his death, my friend LeRoy Stegeman was thinking of others and protecting the planet. The year he celebrated his hundredth birthday, he died. His obituary called for contributions to an environmental science scholarship fund at the university where he taught for so many years.

A father, grandfather and great-grandfather who had buried two wives, Roy rose valiantly over his own infirmities, his hearing loss the most frustrating. He would often hand me a letter during the coffee hour at church. The other day, I found a card with a violet taped to it, simply reading, "A Posey for a Lady." I remember Roy giving it to me.

A zoologist, he was a great lover of the natural world, and enjoyed reminding others of its beauty and our role as stewards. A writer, he wrote three booklets entitled *Life as I See It.*

Under the glass top of my desk, I have another note from Roy, this one on red cardinal stationery: "One can only maintain ability by not overworking it."

Every so often, my eye is drawn to Roy's words and I take them in. It's funny, but the older I get, the more I cherish the advice. I like to believe that the older I get the more I listen to Roy.

The world-renowned analyst Carl Jung wrote:

> A human being would certainly not grow to be seventy or eighty years old if this longevity had not meaning for the species to which he belongs. The afternoon of human life must also have a significance of its own and cannot be merely a pitiful appendage to life's morning.

Having known and loved Roy, I know of the significance of the afternoon of human life. For those in doubt, just listen to the LeRoy Stegemans around you.

TODAY: *Listen for significance.*

When I'm An Old Lady

When I'm an old lady, I'll live with my son, and make his life happy and filled with such fun. I want to pay back all the joy he's provided, returning each deed. Oh, he'll be so excited.

when I'm an old lady and live with my son. I'll write on the wall with red, white, and blue; and bounce on the furniture wearing my shoes. I'll drink from the carton and then leave it out. I'll stuff all the toilets and oh, he will shout.

when I'm an old lady and live with my son. When he's on the phone and just out of reach, I'll get into things like sugar and bleach. Oh, he'll snap his fingers and then shake his head, and when he is done I'll hide under the bed.

when I'm an old lady and live with my son. When my son's wife cooks dinner and calls me to meals, I'll not eat my green beans or salads congealed. I'll gag on my okra, spill milk on the table, and when she gets angry, run fast as I'm able.

when I'm an old lady and live with my son. I'll sit close to the TV, thru the channels I'll click. I'll cross both my eyes to see if they stick. I'll take off my socks and throw one away, and play in the mud until the end of the day.

when I'm an old lady and live with my son. And later, in bed, I'll lay back and sigh, and thank God in prayer and then close my eyes; and my son will look down with a smile slowly creeping, and say with a groan, "she's so sweet when she's sleeping."

when I'm an old lady and live with my son.

—Mary Ann Hopkins

TODAY: *Look forward to being old!*

Writers and artists have long used water to portray life.

To find the common bond between the world's religions, we have the image of the well. All faiths drop their buckets into the same well, separately drawing out their truths. Though we consider ourselves very different, we all drink from the same source.

Rivers can easily be compared to the experience of life. Rivers can't stay still, nor can canoes floating on them. If we try to stay still in the river, we quickly exhaust ourselves treading water, using valuable energy to stay put. Even more fatiguing are efforts to go back. Swimming upstream puts us against the current, and makes the journey a fight. Metaphorically, when we are resisting the current, we are unable to accept the present. The current—the present—is the moment we live in.

The secret, in life and canoeing, is to let go of our fear of moving forward, of the present. Once we are able to trust the river of life, our journey becomes close to effortless. We go with the flow.

TODAY: *Go with the flow.*

As early as colonial times, local governments took responsibility for the poor, not only through subsidies but also through a variety of institutional programs such as almshouses, orphanages and poor farms. State and local governments were responsible for providing care to mentally ill, blind and chronically ill of all ages. America's solution to poverty and other social problems has historically been institutionalization.

Between 1910 and 1970, the proportion of the elderly residing in institutions increased 267 percent. In 1910, about 80,000 older Americans lived in mental institutions or almshouses.

After World War II, the public poorhouses evolved into nursing homes, as they were primarily full of old people. By the 1960s, what we now know as the long-term care institution was born, with the creation of Medicaid. Almshouses were all closed by the 1970s, with 1.1 million older Americans living in institutions, close to 73 percent in nursing homes and 10 percent in mental institutions.

Since 1910, women and men of compassion have worked in thousands of institutions, caring for the frail among us. Poor working conditions, too much to do, too little pay and minimal public awareness were the common experiences of these caregivers. Fortunately, every generation has produced a band of servants, whom we will never be able to adequately thank.

Today there are three times more nursing homes than general hospitals and consequently more patient beds and days spent in nursing homes than hospitals.

What makes institutional life warm and tolerable is the staff. Despite the patients' condition or prognosis, or even their ability to pay, caregivers minister to each individual. Getting to know the full lives and interests of residents, these gentle helpers among us transform the oft-dreaded institutions into home.

TODAY: *Make a home.*

A friend of mine came over last month for a pampering day. She is in her mid-forties, with two adopted babies, ages 16 and 21 months. Both she and her husband work full-time jobs. Understand why I invited her for a pampering day?!

We had our wonderful masseuse Sylvia come to the house, served a good lunch and insisted Sally take a hot bath and then a nap.

Before she went home to her family, we talked about the pressures of being a working mother, and about being a woman in America. She told me about a relative, "The poor thing, she is so concerned about her body and her shape. Last winter, she spent $17,000 on a complete body liposuction. Tummy, hips and bottom."

"$17,000! Did her insurance cover it?" I gasped.

"No, and the worst part is, she has already gained back all 50 pounds."

That we are not our bodies, or perhaps, more accurately, that we are much more than our bodies, is a lesson many women never learn. We have been conditioned by Barbie dolls and Disney cartoons that women are gorgeous, slim, long-legged and forever young.

Author Barbara Walker writes:

> Signs of old womanhood are not supposed to be seen. Women are socially and professionally handicapped by wrinkles and gray hair in a way that men are not. A multi-billion dollar 'beauty' industry exploits women's well-founded fear of looking old. This industry spends megafortunes to advertise elaborately packaged, but mostly useless, products by convincing women that their natural skins are unfit to be seen in public. Every female face must be resurfaced by a staggering variety of colored putties, powders and pastes.
>
> Instead of aging normally though their full life cycle, women are constrained to create an illusion that their growth process stops in the first decade or two of adult-

hood. There is an enormous gulf between a society like this and earlier matriarchal societies where elder women were founts of wisdom, law, healing skills and moral leadership. Their wrinkles would have been badges of honor, not shame.

If we are fortunate to live a long life, we must come to realize that no amount of makeup or surgery can completely erase the hands of time. Rather than resist this truth, a well-adjusted woman embraces it. We are what we are!

TODAY: *See badges of honor.*

Bath time is bliss time for me, and I know I am not alone. Consider all of the flourishing bath businesses, from hot spring spas to body and bath stores. We are 70 percent water, so surely being submerged in a soothing warm bath, like the ones our mothers carried us in, makes us feel complete.

Doug was a bath man himself, well aware of the relaxing qualities of a bath or a shower. "That's why I think we need to do something about the drains in the shower room," Doug said during a discussion with other staff on ways to improve their facility.

"Go into shower room two and smell the drain. Just smell it," he asked his coworkers. Sure enough, a horrible odor of sulfur or sewage was strong in the room, escaping from the drains. Maintenance determined the drains could be blocked with decaying tree roots, or possibly some sewer gasses were traveling back into the facility.

More than 75 people work in the building with Doug, and I would guess 30 of them regularly enter shower room two. Highly tuned in to his residents' well-being, he was the first associate to notice the bad smells in the bath. "This is their time to relax and feel good," he said, "We can't be bringing them into a stinky bathroom!"

Healthcare providers can write job descriptions 24 hours a day, but they will never be able to capture on paper the commitment and dedication Doug brings to the workplace. He so fully relates to those in his care, in some ways, he becomes them. Blessed be this gentle man and all those of his kind.

TODAY: *Become those in your care.*

Touring an impressive new nursing home, funded by a large bequest, Margaret began to compare it to her modest facility and became embarrassed.

"This is like a aircraft carrier! They have everything. It's huge!" Margaret's place was an old Victorian home, the tiny elevator able to carry only one person at a time.

"Look! Everything is new! They even have a chapel with stained glass windows," she continued. After a while, Margaret got quiet. Over lunch, she asked one question. "Where are your animals? I guess we haven't met your pets yet?"

"Oh, we aren't going to have any animals here! This is a sub-acute facility," the administrator said firmly. "We want to maintain a state-of-the-art atmosphere. After all, you would never see dogs or cats in a hospital environment. That's amateur. And who wants to clean up after them? It's just more you-know-what, if you'll pardon the expression."

Driving home, Margaret reviewed her envy. "Maybe I'm crazy, but I think pets make a place feel more like home. We aren't a hospital, we're a home," she thought to herself. "If that makes me an amateur, so be it."

Those of us who have worked in health care know that the latest in bricks and sticks does not make care warmer or better. Amateurs do.

Yes, amateurs. The word comes from the Latin "amare," to love. Give me loving amateurs any day. Especially if they purr when they sit in my lap.

TODAY: *Long live the amateurs!*

A granite quarry reopened in Sheffield, the next town over, and the debate surrounding the resumption of blasting nearly caused a civil war. The quarry had been abandoned for more than 50 years, when suddenly an investor decided there was granite in them thar hills.

Sheffield is a quiet little village, and the only business I've seen there is a pheasant farm. It is also home to our former state poet, a man who has lived and written at his farm for more than 40 years. Writing poetry with dynamite exploding in the distance doesn't work. Mozart or birds chirping make much better background music.

Living in a nursing home, it is staggering how much unwanted noise one must accept. I once tried to take a nap in a California nursing home that had a large flock of parrots. The constant cawing made me crazy! When I went out into the hall to ask someone what that incessant noise was (it sounded like a wind-up toy) I was met with a blank face, "What noise?"

We get used to those noises. Families living close to the train tracks learn to stop talking while the freight cars rumble by. City folks pause their conversations to accommodate the sirens. We adapt.

Sometimes, though, we expect residents of institutions to accept too much. Like the grinding water cooler in a dining room I visited recently. The thing cycled once a minute, a loud whirring sound that made talking impossible. Or the call bell system I endured in a Vermont facility. Surely there was a volume control somewhere!

Few of us are writing poetry, but we still desire a quiet and pleasant atmosphere where we live. In the midst of the hubbub, listen for the noises that can be reduced. Work toward creating a place where you could sleep through the night.

TODAY: *Create more quiet.*

P.S. So far, infrequent and highly muffled blasting seems to be keeping the peace in Sheffield.

Anyone who works as a caregiver is pretty certain his or her job is harder than anyone else's. I've yet to meet a single soul in health care who says, "I don't have enough to do."

Certified nursing assistants and others who provide primary care are often tempted to compare themselves to those sitting behind a desk. "They've got it easy, staring into a computer screen and doing paperwork all day. I'd like to change jobs with them for one day!"

Maybe you should. A job exchange, even for half a day, would be good for all parties. I recommended this activity to a facility where the new administrator was facing a mutiny, almost solely due to his time at the computer.

"He doesn't know anyone's name! He never comes out of there! He even eats in front of the blasted thing!"

I spent a few days in the home, and I made a point of learning what was going on in the administrator's office. It saddened me.

The young fellow had taken over a difficult situation. The building was leased, yet he wasn't provided a copy of the lease. There were no thermostats, and the refrigerator had to be replaced. The phantom lease required the tenant to pay for all upkeep and property maintenance.

He didn't just sit behind the computer during the day. He was there at night, too.

"I'm trying to figure out how I can give them all a raise," he told me in confidence one afternoon. "I've got to do so many repairs, but these people deserve to be paid more."

What a thankless job! Sitting behind a computer, making the numbers work, being a pawn of a larger system that wishes to punish healthcare providers who dare to make a profit. Shame on us.

TODAY: *Understand someone else's job.*

For years the staff had complained about the run-down condition of their nursing home. "Look at those ceiling tiles!" they would point, shaking their heads at the ugly yellow water stains. "And that old flooring. Will they ever clean this place up?"

The sad truth was that their state paid less than almost any other state Medicaid program for the care of residents. The facility's owners were paid less than $80 a day and eking out a living, proud to meet payroll and keep the electricity on.

One happy day a creative nursing assistant arrived with some of his own hanging plants. "We've got to dress up this dining room!" he announced. His coworkers were speechless. "He's bringing his own plants from home!" Soon, colorful tablecloths appeared, and vases with silk flowers. One night, someone brought a steamer to take all the wrinkles out of the tablecloths.

This take-charge approach spread to other departments. Activities put up signs, letting visitors know a faster computer was needed: "We would like residents to be able to download their e-mail in less time!"

Moving from simply observing the problem to deciding to solve it is a huge leap. All it takes is one person, moving from reaction to creation.

TODAY: *Decide to solve problems.*

My husband and I both wanted a dog. He wanted to find one by researching breeds and interviewing dog owners. I wanted a dog to walk into our life.

Having moved to the country, we figured we deserved a big dog that would ride around in the truck with us and scare deer from the garden.

At an outdoor church fair, we noticed a gorgeous dog sitting obediently at his master's feet, though hundreds of people were milling around. We did not recognize the breed. "What kind of dog do you have?"

We quickly got on the trail of the Bérneise Mountain Dog, only to learn the breed is fairly rare. Better to take an adult Bérneise through the rescue league than wait for a puppy.

Around 7 PM on a Wednesday night, the volunteer from the nearest Bérneise Rescue League, in Connecticut, called to interview us. Silly us, we thought the call was for us to hear about the dog!

My husband was on the downstairs phone, and I on the upstairs extension. Once we had passed the screening, we talked about the dog.

"Why is it available?" my husband asked.

The dog had been given as a gift by the grandmother to three children who didn't want a dog. Despite these rough beginnings, the dog was a healthy and playful animal, good with children and well-mannered.

As is often the case, the dog's care had fallen to a disgruntled and disinterested mother. Life with the dog wasn't easy, and the final straw had just occurred.

"The mother reached under the buffet to pull the dog out during dinner, and he nipped her. She'd had it and said the dog had to go to another home."

We hung up a few minutes later, as the rescue league representative said she didn't want an answer tonight.

I ran downstairs in excitement, where my husband was shaking his head.

"What's wrong, aren't you excited?" I blurted.

"We don't want that dog!" he said. I looked at his notes; I looked at mine, and burst out laughing.

In small print at the bottom of my page was the word "nips."

In large print, the only word on his page was "BITES."

TODAY: *Compare notes.*

Mary Beth listens to the residents. The activities director, Mary Beth listens for the little things, the passing remarks easily lost in conversation. Because Mary Beth wears two hearing aids, her careful listening is particularly impressive.

I figured out she was a listener while reading the monthly activities calendar. "You do a World War II discussion group," I noticed, "I haven't seen those anywhere before. That's great! What made you think of it?"

"Well, I just listened to the residents, and I realized we had quiet a few veterans of the Second World War living here. So we started the discussion group."

A few weeks later, I was in another facility waiting for bingo to begin. Someone said "New Orleans" during a conversation. Robert piped up, "I lived in Orleans, Vermont."

I felt like a Mary Beth clone. "Where did you live in Orleans?" I asked.

"On the second floor, above the senior citizen's center. I used to fish out my window!" For the next few minutes, Robert told us all about the sunfish, perch and other fish he caught leaning out his apartment window. I asked if he had fished in the brook behind the nursing home. No, he hadn't. But wouldn't that be a good activity later in the spring?

TODAY: *Listen for the little things.*

It was 5 AM at Chicago's O'Hare Airport, and I felt like a nurses' aide. Specifically, I felt how good it feels to care for others.

My adventure began the day before when, while flying from Savannah to Cleveland, I was grounded by bad weather in Chicago. The airline kept trying to get us back in the air. Flights to Cleveland were scheduled and cancelled for 4:30 PM, 6:30 PM, 9:30 PM and midnight. At 1:30 AM, we were told the next attempt wouldn't be until 6:30 AM.

Before my hopes were dashed, I had given away the dinner coupon supplied by the airline. I wasn't hungry and the young man sitting near me said he was starving. However, by midnight I was ready for something, and even fast food smelled good. I approached the desk and asked for another meal ticket.

"No one is serving food this late," the tired clerk told me, "You'll have to use this for breakfast."

Resigned, I curled up on the airport floor with blankets and a pillow taken from the plane and willed myself to sleep. About four hours later, I woke and surveyed my fellow passengers, crumpled, wrinkled and twisted in and under chairs. Three children snored quietly under a big winter coat on the floor. An older couple clung to each other in frightened sleep. I remembered them; they were trying to get home to Germany.

"Bethany," I thought to myself, "You have been so selfish! Look at these poor folks, so much worse off than you are. You don't have children to be worried about; you aren't flying overseas. You just have a workshop to lead in four hours in Cleveland. Stop feeling sorry for yourself."

I freshened up and got in the McDonald's line. Gee, I thought, it would be neat to surprise the sleeping people with breakfast. I would be the nurses' aide, waking everyone up with juice and coffee.

"Ma'am, do you know this voucher is for $140?" the sleepy McDonald's cashier asked.

Somehow, while I was amazed, I wasn't surprised. "In that case, I would like coffee, juice, danishes and a few yogurts for the people sleeping at gate 15." I enlisted a pilot to help me carry the morning picnic.

"Oh my! Are you a Girl Scout? Are you an angel? Thank you!" And to top it off, I was given a first class seat and made it to Cleveland on time!

TODAY: *Trust the Universe to provide.*

April: Blessed are those who hunger and thirst for righteousness, for they shall be satisfied.

Our physical cravings hold us in great sway, governing both conscious and unconscious actions. We are well acquainted with these powerful urges to satisfy the senses. But what about cravings for justice and integrity?

At the dawn of the Third Millennium, there are 1.2 billion people living in poverty on Planet Earth. Hearing of such need, we automatically experience an inner imbalance and disharmony. Our experience of world justice is like sitting on a teeter-totter: without the other seated and fully sharing the resources, what's the point? How can we enjoy the life ride, knowing others have little or nothing?

Hungry for good, we create ways to motivate ourselves to do right and see the best in our fellow man. Thirsting for righteousness, we encourage others to be virtuous, to make our shared environment a good place to live, marked by fairness and equity.

In the workplace, the righteous caregiver is known for a positive attitude. S/he does not operate out of a sense of righteous indignation, telling others "I've been wronged" or "I've been hurt" or "I'm gonna get mine." These tenacious individuals know that alone they have no righteousness, that only in working together with mutual high standards is it possible to feel satisfied.

When one works up a hunger to give, personal peace comes through obeying the call to love. Aware of the needs of others, such caregivers reach inside for strength, and outside to serve. Leading with conviction, they satisfy their hunger for right living, and feed others in the process.

"I know of no more encouraging fact than the unquestionable ability of man to elevate his life by conscious endeavor."

—Henry David Thoreau

Appreciating the unlimited expressions of conscious endeavor is great fun! Some people choose to take classes or work on a degree. Others develop a new skill, such as massage therapy or rug hooking. We all have curiosities and interests: the secret is to pay attention to these desires and respond to the hunger. Following this inner desire, we are always greatly surprised by unexpected benefits and joys.

Valerie Cooper, a certified nursing assistant from Birmingham, Alabama, is a Native American healer known as Bull Star. Many of her weekends are devoted to Powwows, where she meets with other Indians for celebration and healing.

Among Valerie's gifts is the ability to write poetry, a conscious endeavor that has brought her the great respect of coworkers and family. Writing is also one of her favorite and most successful ways of dealing with work-related stress. Sharing her poems with others, Valerie is able to gently communicate a powerful message of love and kindness, a vision of a beautiful, harmonious world. Reading her work, other caregivers have taken up poetry as well.

Our Elder Voices

> Listen
> Can you hear their voices?
> The voices of our elders.
> Slow down
> Smell the flowers,
> Hear the stories.
> The stories the elders tell.
> Listen
> Can you really hear what they have to say?
> It is not impossible
> It is necessary for our well-being
> Yours and mine

Listen
Hear the stories of their lives
About their family and friends
Slow down and hear their stories.
Listen to the Elder Voices.

—Valerie (Bull Star) Cooper, CNA

TODAY: *Elevate yourself with a conscious endeavor.*

Carpe Rem.

Directly to the right of the church entrance, the sign read "Carpe Rem." I knew "Carpe Diem," seize the day. But what was "Carpe Rem?" Seize what?

I combed my limited Latin for "Rem." "Seize what?" I wondered.

Vermont is the only state that licenses aides; the rest of the nation offers certification. I don't have a problem with being licensed instead of certified. My issue is with the term "nursing assistant." "Nursing assistant?" Hardly. These professionals aren't assisting nurses. They are running the whole show—not supporting actors but lead players. If they are assisting anyone, it is the patient, not the nurse. Nursing assistants hunger and thirst for righteousness, only satisfied when they have done all they can do.

Driving home, my mind returns to the "Carpe Rem" sign. I laugh when the words finally make sense.

Not associated with the church, the broken sign was propped up by the paint and home decorating shop next door. When new, it read "Carpet Remnants."

"Seize the remnants!" I sing to myself. Seize whatever is left of the day, of life, of the patients' lives.

The fragile wisps of women in my care are indeed remnants. Tissue-paper thin. Like milkweed seeds, they would blow away if the blankets were removed. The life force burns in their eyes, peering out through worn-out skin bags, tired shells, holding light from days gone by.

"Seize the remnants!" my heart sings. Clutch their sweetness, their dearness, their preciousness. Hold on tight, and learn life's secrets. Be taught compassion, mercy and tenderness. Satisfy cravings to serve and love.

TODAY: *Seize the remnants!*

Managers will say, "If I could only get a few more like Therese, Rhonda and Debra. They'll never leave." Every healthcare institution has its core of long-timers, those incredibly dedicated employees who belong there and will never leave. Working anywhere else, they would feel lost and dissatisfied.

Throughout the world, there is a network of communities called L'Arche homes, built under the leadership of Jean Vanier. Mentally handicapped individuals and their caregivers live in these homes, in the spirit of the Beatitudes. In 1985, Henri J. M. Nouwen, a Catholic priest, author and professor, went to work as a chaplain in the Toronto L'Arche home and wrote this:

> It was interesting to hear the distinction between handicapped people and assistants is becoming less important than the distinction between long-term community members and short-term helpers...those who have built a real and lasting bond with L'Arche are especially responsible for making visitors, short-term assistants and new handicapped people feel welcome.

> So, it is a community, always adapting itself to new people, always open to surprises, always willing to try new things, but with a solid center of committed people who know the importance of permanency.

Become aware of this feeling of community. Who are the members of your solid center, your Royal Family of veteran staff? Thank them for their commitment and dependability.

TODAY: *Appreciate the solid center.*

(Reprinted from *The Road to Daybreak, A Spiritual Journey* by Henri J. M. Nouwen. New York, Doubleday Books. Copyright © 1988 p. 351)

Eating an orange in front of others, most of us have been trained to graciously offer others a slice. I remember in India being scolded for not also offering the peel, as I was in the presence of very hungry people.

To not be satisfied unless others are satisfied is the rule of those who hunger and thirst for righteousness, for uniformly decent conditions. This year, while visiting nursing homes throughout the United States, I was awakened to small inequities that are causing major staff discontent.

Dress codes are the subject, and the problems are caused by an inconsistent enforcement of policy. Although not consciously established to create divisions, dress codes are doing just that.

"Why are the nurses allowed to wear street clothes, and the CNAs are not?" is a question I was asked in the South and Midwest.

Almost as frequently heard is this question, "Why aren't CNAs allowed to use the phone for personal calls when the nurses are?"

The haves and the have-nots. From parking places to coat hooks, from dress codes to phone privileges, the challenge remains the same: for all associates to be treated in a just fashion. If you believe inequities are causing an angry undercurrent among caregivers, please make a decision to work things out. Resist anger and name-calling: look for common ground and common good.

TODAY: *Stand for justice.*

Margaret had left the assisted living facility near Cleveland to work somewhere else. A change of management made her "pack her bags," she recalled.

But like others in the brotherhood and sisterhood of caregivers, Margaret missed the residents. She realized no workplace is perfect, and no boss is always fair. When a position opened up, Margaret decided to apply. She had been away long enough.

"My first day on the job, I heard this commotion at the end of the hall," Margaret smiled. "It was one of my old residents. She was so happy to see me; she was lifting her walker up in the air and banging it on the floor, hooting 'look who's back!' It sure made me feel good."

What I love about this story is the banging walker. So spontaneous, so total, the resident used everything she had in her power and reach to welcome Margaret. Had she been healthier, I bet cartwheels would have occurred!

Few of us realize the impact we have on the lives of others. Margaret had no idea how much she had been loved and missed. Hungering for her residents, she was well satisfied.

TODAY: *Realize your impact.*

Ever have a good idea you wanted others to believe in? In high school, my class of 500 students was preparing for graduation. We were required to pay $10 to buy a paper gown and rented cap for the ceremony.

A disposable gown seemed stupid to me: what a waste of $5,000! I proposed we build a house for a homeless family, which could be done for $5,000 through a special program. "That would show we were really educated, and make our graduation mean something!" I told my teachers and fellow classmates.

But even the principal said the class would miss their pictures in the traditional cap and gown. My suggestion of navy skirts or pants and white tops (our school colors) was dismissed.

For a good idea to become realized, other people must support it. The philosopher William James wrote, "The community stagnates without the impulse of the individual; the impulse dies away without the sympathy of the community."

In your facility, while there are standard and proven procedures for much of what you do, new ideas are still important. Every so often, someone will see something differently and daily operations are improved. I joke about the shoes everyone wears at Maple Lane Nursing Home in Barton. Clogs were in when I trained. Today, feet are clad in suede slip-ons, all because the new Director of Nursing, Sue Brown, was wearing some when she took the job.

Among you there are idea people, who need the sympathy of the community, support and encouragement. Before you say, "I like the old way," pay attention.

TODAY: *Support new ideas.*

Some people seem to know what they will do with their lives from Day One. Perhaps they are born into a family of caregivers, as were the six sisters I met in Wisconsin who work as nurses' aides in the same facility!

Mike Brown's mother took him to visit nursing homes when he was a boy. It was then he chose a career in long-term care; he just knew. Many of us aren't as fortunate, and test drive several careers before we find one that grabs us. Discerning what we want to do is critical, and it can help to hear the observations of others.

The scientist Charles Darwin didn't have the slightest idea that he possessed a talent for science until he was a young man at Cambridge University. There, he received powerful encouragement from his professor of botany, John Henslow. Henslow persuaded Darwin he had talent, and nominated him as the candidate for scientist on the voyage of the Beagle. We remember that Darwin's primary research for his pioneering work, *The Origin of the Species*, was based on data collected during the five year voyage of the Beagle. Describing the role this trip played in his life, Darwin referred to it as a rebirth.

Seeing strengths and talent in others, it is wise to acknowledge and encourage. Caregivers are in high demand. Wherever you see the raw ingredients needed to become a dedicated servant, follow Professor Henslow's lead. Encourage talent and invite candidates to visit your facility. Why not pull together a world-class crew? You may just experience a rebirth.

TODAY: *Encourage others to care.*

Words of gratitude for caregivers, from two residents of St. Patrick's Residence, Naperville, Illinois:

> You are the grandest person I've ever seen. You gently, patiently encourage me. 'Now put one leg down, now the next. You are doing fine.' This makes me feel good and makes me want to do anything you tell me, even though it hurts. You push me on. I'm willing to try anything with you.

> When I know you're working, I don't even worry about getting stockings on, my brace and hearing aides. Those are the three things I worry about in the morning. 'Who is going to do this for me?' When you're here, I'm real at ease. You are wonderful.

Remember that childhood song, "Home, Home on the Range?" My favorite line is, "Where never is heard a discouraging word." As these residents report, your encouraging words make all the difference in their days and lives. Think about your importance: someone will try anything you tell her to do. Someone else actually stops worrying when you walk in the room. Your presence leads to courage.

Your strength of character and loving sense of what is right are appreciated and persuasive. On those days you question your work and worth, think of this power. Residents need your encouraging words.

TODAY: *Encourage resident courage.*

When I was a lobbyist, I called it my Power Whine. When I was two years old, my mother called it a tantrum.

The art of convincing others of our position is delicate business. The finest persuaders around us are politicians, preachers, and salespeople.

Working with people, you spend your whole day respectfully striving to get others to do what is best for them. Mr. Martin doesn't want to get up. Alice will not lie down. Mrs. Bean is afraid of that bathtub.

You cajole, joke, compromise, and even distract residents to get results. Mature caregivers know what needs to be done. Your desire is to serve the resident, making him as comfortable as possible. And when this happens, your satisfaction is great.

Insecure people are rarely able to persuade. Instead, they may throw a fit, refuse to speak or walk out. Coworkers might mistakenly interpret these actions as those of spoiled brats or prima donnas. But what makes a person use these immature techniques?

When people believe they are powerless and have no voice—that no one will listen to them—they turn to dramatics: issuing ultimatums, throwing fits or falling silent.

To outgrow such game playing, we must become more certain of our beliefs. Focusing on doing the right thing and living up to our words, we can grow and become more confident. And here's the best part of the equation: once we believe in ourselves, the rest of the world will follow.

TODAY: *Believe in yourself.*

My father never has believed in the communication gap. When my room was mess, he communicated his feelings clearly: the vacuum was placed under my covers. Truly my father's daughter, I communicated my lack of desire to clean with equal precision: I slept with the vacuum.

Living and working with others, finding that fine line between nagging and reminding takes diplomacy. Dinah the Diplomat has mastered walking that line.

Dinah had been disheartened by the performances of some of her colleagues, particularly the younger aides. "They just don't respect the old people, and it has bothered me." Rather than sounding bossy or judgmental, Dinah decided to motivate without criticizing. Tracing her hand in a thumb's up position, she cut out several dozen hands and wrote little cheerful quotes and verses on them. Every few days, she secretly hung up different hands on the staff bathroom stall doors.

"Who's the thumbs-up angel?"

"Did you see that funny one about gossiping?"

Dinah's gentle, positive touch continues. She has expanded to putting up posters and pictures by the time clock. And she's added a few other communication angels to her team. By example and with love, Dinah is softening the hearts of coworkers, and teaching the important lesson of respecting others.

TODAY: *Communicate diplomatically.*

Florence Nightingale, the founder of nursing, came from a wealthy family that forbade her to enter a caregiving career.

By the mid-1800s, caring for the sick and dying was no longer considered a holy vocation, having been removed from the hands of the priests and nuns by King Henry VIII. Drunks and prostitutes were the only women working in Europe's early hospitals, and Florence would disgrace her parents by taking such a job.

But Florence's heart drew her to the work. At age 17, she said, "God spoke to me and called me to His Service." She refused marriage proposals and talked only of nursing, pleading with her parents to let her follow her inner light, which clearly directed her to caring. Hoping to distract their eldest daughter from such nonsense, the Nightingales sent her on more than one long boat trip down the river Nile.

In her early twenties, Florence asked family friend Samuel Gridley Howe, an American philanthropist, "Would it be a 'dreadful thing' if I were to devote my life to nursing?"

Mr. Howe replied, "Not a dreadful thing at all. I think it would be a very good thing." It would be unusual—and in England anything unusual was regarded as unsuitable—but he encouraged her to, "Go forward...act up to your inspiration and you will find there is never anything unbecoming or unladylike in doing your duty for the good of others."

Nearly 10 years later Florence's hunger for service won out and she began her lifelong career in nursing. She would become the world expert on the design of hospitals and on sanitation in India. She would also create the first system to classify causes of death. Of her work Florence wrote:

> Nursing is an Art; and if it is to be made an art, requires an exclusive devotion, as hard a preparation as any painter's or sculptor's work; for what is having to do with dead canvas or cold marble compared with having to do with the living body—the temple of God's spirit. It is one of the Arts; I have almost said, the finest of the Fine Arts.

Many of us have faced similar struggles in being certain about beginning a career as a caregiver. Family members worry about tiring schedules, draining emotional duties and poor compensation. We must remain confident and strong, feeling blessed to answer the call for the good of others.

TODAY: *Answer the call with strength and confidence.*

(Reprinted from *Letters and Reflections*. Ed. by Monica Furlong. Evesham, UK, Arthur James Ltd. Copyright © 1996 p. 64.)

Toni Tollestrup, a woman of great talent, has worked in many settings, including as a nursing assistant in California. Serving on Beverly Healthcare's National CNA Leadership Council, Toni shared her favorite motivational book, Elwood Chapman's *Attitude: Your Most Priceless Possession.*

"This little book has helped me more than anything else I've ever read," Toni told the Council. More than one million copies of the book have been published!

Professor Chapman's book is based on a 50-minute lecture he delivered in various forms for more than 30 years to hundreds of organizations. During post-lecture discussions "the one question asked most often was, 'How can I stay positive?'" The book answers this question.

> My experience has taught me that attitude is a highly personal and sensitive topic. No one can force a change in your personal attitude. You alone have that responsibility, and you must do it your own way.

> An excellent starting place in your quest to stay positive is to examine your present attitude. I suggest being honest, but not too serious, because too much introspection could cause you to lose your perspective and or your sense of humor...which could be counterproductive.

To keep readers smiling, the author includes some of his amoeba drawings.

Amoeba drawings? Amoebas divide in two every hour.

> This may be a signal that the best way for humans to keep a positive attitude is to constantly renew it by sharing it with others.

TODAY: *Share your positive attitude with others and watch it divide and grow like an amoeba!*

When we get sick, what does it mean?

Usually we say we're run down, children brought germs from school or that our immunity is damaged. Why else do we get sick? In my adult life, I have been sick just a few times. Looking at each incident, I can see my illnesses began in my mind.

In 1976, I got my first job as a reporter at the *Adrian Daily Telegram* in Adrian, Michigan. Editor of my junior and senior high school newspapers, with a bachelor's degree in journalism from the University of Michigan and two years of college-level journalism teaching behind me, I didn't feel nervous; I felt excited. But I began to have diarrhea, and it didn't clear up. Concerned, I went to the doctor.

"I used to play football," the doctor said. "And before every game, I would go behind the bleachers and throw up." Why is he telling me this?

"If it hasn't cleared up after your first paycheck, come back and see me." What a wise man. I didn't go back.

In 1982 I was divorced. Like most divorces, it was rugged and had taken close to a year to resolve. Never had I been through such a stressful, painful and lonely experience. I had to be strong and my family was many states away. The day following the final hearing, I became violently ill with the flu. I was feverish, nauseous, and slept for four days.

Knowing stress can make me sick, I've learned to take better care of myself, drink lots of water, get exercise and plenty of sleep.

Take a moment and look at your ailments. Back trouble? What in the past is still bothering you? What is holding you back? Stomach trouble? What anger are you holding on to? What do you need to let go of?

Our minds and bodies are one; we've just decided to separate them. Take care of your well-being, reconnect and pay attention to your needs.

TODAY: *Reconnect your mind and body.*

I received this quote, attributed to Kathleen Fischer, on a birthday card: "Hope is an act of collaboration, it cannot be achieved alone. We offer grains or fragments of hope to one another so that everyone's sense of possibility can grow. In this way we can do together what might seem impossible alone."

Therese, an aide for 10 years, told me about the Sunday morning one of her residents, Mrs. La Flam, said she didn't want to change rooms. A new admission had started the dominoes falling, and Mrs. La Flam was told she had to move to a different wing and be assigned a new roommate. Having heard this on Friday, Mrs. La Flam considered it for days, and asked Therese if she could talk with her a minute. "Is there a policy that I must move here, even if I don't want to?" she asked Therese. "You see, I am content here, and I don't wish to move. Can they make me?" Mrs. La Flam then began to cry.

Therese recalled the severe depression Mrs. La Flam suffered at admission, and how hard the aides had worked to help her pull out of it. She decided to talk with a few other aides and with the charge nurse.

The opinion was unanimous: Mrs. La Flam was doing well, and a move didn't seem in her best interest. Presenting the case to the charge nurse, Therese was careful to point out she was reporting Mrs. La Flam's opinions, and that she was doing so at Mrs. La Flam's request. The staff was in support.

After listening to the case, the charge nurse told Therese she agreed, and would tell the director of nursing on Monday that everyone had agreed the move was not a good idea.

"I felt so good!" Therese said later. "I was an advocate for my resident. I had cried with Mrs. La Flam when she talked with me, but when I went to the nurse, I didn't get emotional. I made my point and it worked!"

TODAY: *Advocate for your residents.*

My husband teases me that I am a multi-track player, and he is a one-track. "You can listen to the radio, be on the phone, type on the computer and follow a conversation in another room at the same time. I can do any of those things, but only one at a time."

I've always felt women could multi-track more easily than men, though I'm not sure why. Certainly motherhood prepares us. Another good training ground is working as a caregiver. Without efficiently performing several tasks at once, the list never gets done.

What about multi-tracking in less obvious ways? How many co-workers and residents can you cheer up in one workday? How often can you pass a smile or a wink to a waiting face?

My friend Dorothy told me about the day that, as an education major in college, she finally could go observe a classroom. "I had been waiting for five semesters, and at last I could visit a real school and watch kids learn. I was so excited. I knew I was one step closer to being a teacher."

Seeing Dorothy at the door, the teacher said, "Look, I'm having a bad day, so don't expect anything. In fact, I can't handle any questions. Just sit over there."

Hearing Dorothy's disappointed voice as she told the story, I looked into my own life and wondered if I had let down others who had been waiting for opportunities. I recalled this saying: "A candle loses nothing by lighting another candle."

Before we carry a grouchy attitude into work, we should think a minute. Who has been waiting to see you? What does this day mean to them? Can you light another candle?

TODAY: *Light candles.*

The founding fathers of this country were great practitioners of charity. Long before the United Way or Red Cross existed, individuals and families willingly gave to others.

George Washington was typical in this respect:

> Even while leading the military struggle against Great Britain, he could not neglect his obligation. In November 1774 he wrote a letter to the agent of his estate at Mt. Vernon that stressed, in effect, an open house:

> Let the hospitality of the house, with respect to the poor, be kept up. Let no one go away hungry. If any of this kind of people shall be in want...supply their necessities...; and I have no objection to your giving my money in charity...What I mean by having no objection is that my desire is that it should be done.

Reading the incomes of political candidates reported in the press, I have been surprised by their limited tithing—way below the customary 10 percent. With millions of dollars in income, they give little.

I offset this image with the giving patterns of Vermont state employees I have known. One Christmas, I was delivering cookies to the bookkeepers and accountants who staff the Medicaid rate-setting division. As we talked about holiday preparations, Jimmy Reardon said he was shopping for his adopted family that night.

"Adopted family?" I asked.

"Yeah. We got names of needy families and a list what they need."

Great men like George Washington and Jimmy Reardon set an example for us all. Let none of us have any objection to giving to charity.

TODAY: *Give to others.*

(Reprinted with the permission of The Free Press, a Division of Simon & Schuster, Inc., from *From Poor Law to Welfare State: A History of Social Welfare in America* by Walter I. Trattner. Copyright © 1974, 1979, 1984, 1989 by The Free Press. Copyright © 1994, 1998 by Walter I. Trattner.)

Hope you got your taxes in! Makes me long for the good old days—that is, before 1913.

America's federal income tax didn't begin until 1913. Without taxes, few government programs existed. And, as programs have increased over the decades, so have taxes.

1965 was a big year, with the creation of two federal health programs, Medicare and Medicaid. Medicare is all federal tax dollars, and used by those over 65 years of age or younger and disabled. Medicaid is a combination of federal and state tax dollars, and targets low-income Americans.

Medicaid is the primary payer of bills in nursing homes, as most folks do not have enough savings to cover their nursing home stay. At this writing, $90 billion Medicaid dollars are spent annually in nursing homes.

Want a raise?

Want your taxes to go up?

See the problem? Nursing home staff deserves to earn a living wage, yet no one wants higher taxes. Until long-term care insurance is more widely purchased, nursing homes will continue to be full of patients who live their final years on welfare.

By understanding the funding of long-term care in this country, caregivers can become advocates for the purchase of long-term care insurance. Americans need to take personal responsibility for the financing of their long-term care. If we don't, we will continue to ask caregivers to pay for our poor planning by working for less than adequate wages.

TODAY: *Advocate for personal responsibility.*

Lance Youles' high school experiences as a nursing home volunteer and nurse's aide led him to a career in long-term care, which has included working in elite private-pay as well as inner-city facilities. He has owned and operated homes, been a state regulator, worked for national companies and even cared for his own family members.

With more than 21 years in the business of caring for America's elders, Lance Youles has developed some powerful teaching tools for communicating the right way to serve those most in need.

Reading his site, www.ismi.net/lryteach, I found lots of resources and inspiration. As a writer, I am especially excited by discussions around language and its influence. In describing the healthy nursing homes of the future, Mr. Youles writes that the conventional thinking of yesterday must evolve into the progressive thinking of tomorrow:

> out with good intentions (process thinking)—in with results (outcome thinking)
> out with boss—in with coach
> out with treating residents—in with serving them
> out with facility—in with community
> out with resident rooms—in with households
> out with skilled units—in with aging in place.

If you haven't spent any time thinking about the power of words, do so. While it is easy to dismiss Mr. Youles' distinctions, saying, "they're just words," please resist. Ever notice how you get a lot more respect on the phone when you refer to yourself as doctor? Or what it feels like to be told to "shut up!" Words have great power to shape our opinions and behavior.

Sit down at the next staff meeting and talk about your own list of words that are ready to be traded in. Why not start with the terms "feeder" and "probation?"

TODAY: *Watch your words.*

American youth aged 8 to 17 continue to say that TV commercials and other types of advertising influence their purchase decisions, according to the 2000 Roper Youth Report, an annual syndicated research study focused on American kids, tweens and teens, released in January 2001.

The 250-page report explores the mood of young Americans and their growing optimism. It examines their developing sense of self, the elements nurturing that identity, and their interactions with family and friends.

Written to assist companies better market to this age group, the study can also help those of us who wish to attract young people to human services and helping professions.

The top-ranked dreams of this age group are:

Being rich-56%; Traveling the world-43%; Being famous-43%; Being smarter-40% Being a great athlete-40%; Seeing my future-38%; Helping other people-37%. (Copyright 2001, USA TODAY. Reprinted with permission.)

I was initially discouraged that being rich was the top dream and helping others at the bottom. But compared to the 1995 results of the same survey, I was heartened. Helping others grew by six percent in this year's study, and being rich dropped by nine percent.

The influence of forces outside the family on youth is obvious. I doubt parents are preaching that, above all, they want their sons and daughters to be rich. That message comes from the world of entertainment, where we idealize and worship celebrities.

Where are the competing voices, speaking of the great satisfaction that comes from helping others, from satisfying our own desire to do right? Most of these voices are busy serving others in nursing homes, hospitals, schools, mental health clinics, soup kitchens and other places of compassion. All together now: speak up!

TODAY: *Influence children's choices.*

I firmly believe no one consciously decides to go to work and have a bad day. Yet many of us do.

> How do we break through mounds of negative attitudes and break free to make the uncommon choice for transformation? Why do some people appear to wake up and make this choice, but in a short time return to the sleeping state? Why do others run from one spiritual experience to another, one seminar to another, one religion to another, in a seemingly endless pursuit of transformation?

> What is the secret element that causes some people to make the uncommon choice and tenaciously move through all obstacles towards..wholeness and holiness? The secret lies in each person's inner commitment to work toward developing positive attitudes toward self, others and life.

I grew up in a family that made judgments. We watched and commented, whether about television or the neighbors' lives. My husband's family did not. Early in our marriage, he repeatedly pointed out my habit of judging, asking why I did it. I honestly had never noticed my behavior. I just did it; it was part of who I was, how I looked at the day. For the past ten years, I have worked at outgrowing the habit.

Being free of the obligation or need to judge, I can be with people in a much different way. I can seek to understand and appreciate them, to enjoy them as they are, not as a project to be evaluated and corrected.

As I write this entry, our news is full of reports on the bloody murder of two professors at nearby Dartmouth College. Last night, two teenage boys were arrested for the crime. I feel such incredible sadness for everyone, the dead and the living. I hear others crying for life in prison for the boys, but something inside me cries back, "No!" Instead, I find myself wondering what went wrong, what we have done to produce a society where teenage murderers are created.

TODAY: *Seek to understand instead of judge.*

After yesterday's talk of judging, I am reminded of one of the kindest men I've ever met. His name was Steve and he wore a disguise.

He disguised himself as a man who didn't care about others. With a wooden expression, he was courteous and punctual and expected the same from others. Steve managed a modestly-sized nursing home in a modestly-sized city. He was a modest man.

The highly emotive and expressive staff, mainly women, believed Steve's disguise was real. They didn't know he was a gentle soul who cared about his employees and residents. They interpreted Steve's shyness as coolness, his reserve as meaning he was the Tin Man—without a heart.

People used expressions like "He's one of a kind," and "He's harmless" to describe Steve.

Before I share the happy ending to this story, let me digress a moment and ask readers to review the conclusions you've drawn about coworkers and managers. Is it possible someone is just too afraid to reveal him or herself to you? Could they need some extra attention or warmth in order to be brought to room temperature? Isn't getting to know someone a two-way street?

Steve went away to a workshop, and when he returned he called his department heads together. "It was amazing," one of the team members said later. "He had hives all over his neck when he talked, but he basically told us he loved us. We couldn't believe it."

TODAY: *Don't fall for disguises.*

Deb was disgusted and there was no hiding it in her note to me:

> If you come to my facility, you'll see the LPNs and RNs sitting behind the counter most of the day supposedly doing paperwork but writing a little here and there in the middle of their conversations. Then you'd see about six CNAs, three up working and three sitting down. Three of us are working our tails off on the floor. The sitting just gets to me.

I remember an experience I had at Currier's General Store a few years ago. Currier's, the one store in my town, was holding a 30th anniversary party. I was asked to volunteer for three days and serve free refreshments. It was exhausting!

Looking around, I realized there were no chairs to sit on. Jim Currier, the shopkeeper, doesn't sit all day, nor do his staff. He provides no chairs, believing there is always something to do.

I suggested to Deb she ask the director of nursing to discuss this issue at a staff meeting. By not trying to lead the discussion herself, Deb could tone down some of her negativity.

Maybe it is time to get some pedometers for everyone's belts that measure how much people have walked in a day. Have a contest, get people moving.

TODAY: *Keep moving.*

Toji Moore is a CNA in Kansas, working at Lincoln East. Following a day-long workshop, Toji decided she wanted to give a talk in her facility. She asked me to help her prepare. In turn, I asked her to e-mail me two points she wanted to talk about and a little story to make her points. Toji wrote:

> 1-I want better communication so everyone can see that no one is doing more work than the next person, and 2-I want them to see that this job is important and that we're not in it for the money. I want them to know you have to have a caring heart and a better understanding of your job.

> My story: We have a resident named Martha. I get off work at 7:00 PM and every evening before I go home I put Martha to bed because she doesn't want anyone else to help her. She says no one does it like me. She likes to be put to bed a certain way and no one else will do it. So I stay over a little to put her to bed and she goes to bed happy and that makes me feel good. When I come back to work after a day off Martha hugs me and tells me she missed me. That's a feeling no one can take from me.

Toji was ready! I suggested that after her talk she could ask the audience to turn to the person next to him or her and tell a story of feeling special or happy.

My only other suggestion was to practice in front of the mirror at home. Honest! The mirror can be much harder than talking to real people (since we're our own harshest critics), so when you do talk, it is feels easier.

TODAY: *Prepare to share some happy stories.*

Discovering another set of wonderful people reaching out to the nursing home community gladdens my heart. Attracting new, caring people into long-term care facilities is a wonderful cause.

Have you visited www.faithfulfriends.org? Faithful Friends is a nursing home ministry led by Larry and Sandy Wasserman of Hobe Sound, Florida. Visitors to the web site are welcomed and encouraged to use "many tools and resources that will aid you in caring for and ministering to the confined elderly in nursing homes."

The Wassermans' mission is to serve the servants, providing encouragement and support to individuals, organized ministries, chaplains, activities directors and staff. Support includes a monthly newsletter, Bible studies, free drawings, links to other caregiving web sites and videos. If you know of family or friends with time to spare, why not contact Faithful Friends and order one of these films to inspire them into volunteering?

"A Song For Grandmother," by Dorothy Miller & Jeremiah Films. This 30-minute video is excellent for recruiting and training new volunteers.

"White Unto Harvest" This 17-minute video from the Sonshine Society presents the Challenge of Nursing Home Ministry. Includes 50 accompanying recruiting leaflets.

"Reaping the Harvest" A two-part, 70-minute video from the Sonshine Society, covering both one-on-one and group ministry in Nursing Homes.

Busy caregivers love volunteers. So do the residents!

TODAY: *Encourage volunteers.*

Oh, if every day could be survey day!

Not because of the stress generated by the presence of inspectors, but because everyone pitches in.

Being on our best behavior when company is present is human nature. But it is also revealing, as we learn just what people are capable of when they make an effort.

At a gathering of administrators from a national nursing home organization, we were discussing some of the snafus that arise during a state or federal survey. When Ed told his story, we all quickly agreed—it was bad:

> I was out there on the floor, helping during lunch. I knew something was wrong, because usually the staff is so appreciative when I feed a resident or offer and extra hand. But this time, they were all giving me dirty looks.

Turns out Ed, the administrator, was feeding a resident who had a G Tube and was not supposed to be swallowing anything. Uh oh.

After the laughter subsided, we talked about how nearly half the people working in nursing homes spend their days writing down what the other half are doing with the residents. Is this really the design government intended when the rules and regulations for nursing homes were written?

Whenever possible, stay where the action is; be with the residents. Resist the call of the desk. Make every day survey day, from your own point of view.

TODAY: *Act like it is survey day.*

Staff turnover is high in all departments, but it seems the stability that once characterized the director of nursing services position is no more.

Among managers, the director of nursing is the lynch-pin in matters of quality. A director of nursing's performance is reflected in the CNA ranks. Nursing homes that lose their director of nursing court disaster: administrators and CNAs follow her out the door, and every measure of quality begins to slide.

Knowing this position is critical to facility performance, why would any company recycle damaged goods?

Misty was not a well-liked or respected director of nursing. Her "Friday night wardrobe," as the staff referred to it, made staff uncomfortable. Her habit of disciplining staff wherever she ran into them was also upsetting, and caused publicly-reprimanded employees to unite against her. Complaints piled up at the home office, and it appeared Misty was on shaky ground. When she was transferred to a sister facility, the staff rejoiced, though they couldn't understand why she was given another job.

Everyone found it easy to understand what happened at the new facility. On the lobby bulletin board, informal pictures of the management team were displayed. The photos were of Misty, the administrator, and department heads, taken at a recent open house. Upon closer inspection, one could see Misty's face had been carefully scratched out of every picture, and replaced with an unflattering term.

Rather than allowing this awful incident to serve as a wake-up call and questioning what she might be doing to generate such anger, Misty went on the warpath. "I'm going to find out who did that and I will have them fired!" she announced.

Good directors of nursing must command and return the respect of staff. Commit yourself to supporting good people in these positions. We can afford no less.

TODAY: *Support good directors of nursing.*

Several times a year I receive giant reports, sometimes weighing more than one pound, on the staffing crisis in long-term care. Such studies are the typically generated by government mandates, foundation grants or academic initiatives.

Several times a week I am contacted by providers, advocates and family members about improving the nursing home environment. We're all talking about it, so what can we do?

Plenty. So much is wrong with the nursing home model as it currently operates; it's hard to identify one starting point. Though it may not be the most critical area needing to be changed, I recommend facilities look at flexible schedules as an idea that will produce immediate positive results.

Yesterday I heard an advertisement on national television, announcing that Ford automobile dealerships now have Saturday hours. For folks who work 9 to 5, five days a week, this news is music! No more arranging with a friend to be taken to work, making sure the day starts early enough so no work is missed.

Our culture is a 24-hour public experience. Most of us have access to a grocery store, gas station and laundromat any time of day or night. Daycare centers are advertising longer and longer hours, some open 24 hours.

Nursing facilities that are offering staff flexible hours experience lower turnover and fewer call-ins. Rather than struggling to find a place to put their children from 6:45 AM until school starts, mothers are hired to start work at 8:30 AM The kids must be especially grateful, with a little more sleep and less hustling. "But we need staff earlier to get people up!" comes the cry of protest.

Another suggestion: let residents wake up when they want to, and forget the crazy hospital morning schedule that doesn't suit a place called HOME. Staff will tell you they much prefer helping someone get ready for the day when she isn't fighting a 6 AM wake-up call. Everyone benefits.

TODAY: *Be flexible.*

Trends in business reveal our culture's values and mores.

The convenience of the 24-hour business mentality comes with a price. Able to work every hour of every day, some of us don't know how or when to stop.

When I moved to Vermont in 1978, few grocery stores were open on Sundays, and the sale of beer and wine was prohibited. Today a store will sell to us whenever we have the money. We have forgotten the concepts of "down time" and being closed.

Expanded hours and an ever-increasing desire for profit means more work hours and more pressure to produce. The United States Department of Agriculture (USDA) poultry processing line speed limit increased from 70 birds per minute in 1979 to 91 per minute in 1999. Sixty percent of the poultry companies surveyed by the Department of Labor were found to be in violation of the Fair Labor Standards Act, and at one plant, violations involving a substantial probability of death or serious injury increased more than 150 percent between 1997 and 1998.

More chickens, more profits, but at what cost to the worker?

In health care and other human services professions, we see more and more employees coming to work sick. So sick they should be at home, recuperating. "Oh, no. I can' t afford to miss work," the employee says. "Oh, no. We need her on the floor," the supervisor adds.

Given that the caregiver's life call is about taking care of health, the irony here is too great! Why are we pushing one another to ignore illness and keep working? Don't we deserve the same consideration as our residents?

Take a moment and review the expectations placed on you by yourself and your employer. Is it time to take a deep breath and promise to take better care of you? Can you allow yourself a needed sick day?

TODAY: *Review expectations.*

How do you say thank you? Like professing one's love, appreciating one another is an opportunity to be creative and clever.

Working in a setting that is rooted in routine, we can fall into a rut when it comes to expressing gratitude.

Wherever I go, caregivers tell me they don't feel appreciated, that they don't hear "thank you" enough. I believe if the facility administrator spent one entire day systematically thanking employees, at the end of the day someone would complain, "She didn't thank me!"

Acknowledging the contributions of staff is not only management's job. If we are truly part of a team, and dedicated to our careers, seeing the good in others is part of what we do. Why wait for someone else to deliver kind words?

Vicki Larson, a care specialist at Beverly Healthcare's Covington Heights facility in Sioux Falls, South Dakota told me about the Thank You Store. The small shop is in the facility and open several hours daily. "We can buy all kinds of cute gifts, like angels and other things to give each other, when we want to thank someone for a good job." The staff suggests the items the Thank You Store will stock.

In Wichita, I visited a nursing home that used another innovative approach. All associates were given a fixed amount of facility play money at the beginning of every week. When they saw an employee do something worthy of notice and gratitude, they would award the person some play money. Facility play money is spent in the home's snack shop. Sodas, candy, chips and other treats are available.

Good caregivers experience great inner satisfaction when a job is well done. When another respected caregiver recognizes our good work, the satisfaction is even sweeter. What new ways can you say thank you?

TODAY: *Say thank you in a new way.*

The Carmelite Sisters of the Aged and Infirm graciously hosted my retreat at Our Lady's Manor in the village of Dalkey, on the East coast of Ireland. The order's Mother-house is in Germantown, NY, also home to the Avila Institute of Gerontology. Their mission is operating nursing homes, 23 in the United States and Our Lady's Manor, near Dublin.

I had my meals in the nursing home that week, attended mass in the facility chapel and was also invited on a building tour. To my surprise, all of the resident rooms on the basement floor were empty.

"We found our patients didn't like the darkness of these rooms," the Sisters explained. Each room had windows, but they faced a brick wall. Moving the residents to vacant upstairs rooms, the nuns seized on an idea. Why not offer basement rooms to staff when they need them?

Several of the basement rooms are regularly used by aides and nurses. Sometimes weather makes it easier to stay overnight at the home rather than risk travel. On other occasions an employee may be between apartments and need temporary housing.

With the census in most nursing facilities in the U.S. dropping, many administrators are trying to figure out what to do with open rooms. Perhaps the Dalkey solution would work. Surely there is no more affordable, clean and convenient shelter for staff! For some single men and women, the right arrangement might be a tremendously attractive benefit.

TODAY: *Provide staff housing.*

May: Blessed are the merciful, for they shall receive mercy.

If you inhale, you shall exhale.

Such is the promise of this Beatitude, that by simply showing mercy one receives mercy. Hospice workers know this lesson well. The literal translation of hospice from the Latin is both "guest" and "host." We cannot imagine this circumstance, to be both the visitor and the householder, yet this is the sacred experience of caring for others. When we are ministering to the needs of another, the reward is ongoing and great. In the giving, we receive. Based on faith and experience, we know we will be given the same measure we give another. When we care for we will be cared for.

Only in resolutely living in mercy, every day, can we expect mercy to be returned. Mercy is a practice, more than a feeling or a sentiment. Mercy is visible in deeds, words, sentiments, prayers and tears. When we make a mistake we want people to forgive us; we want mercy. With mercy, we are forgiven our faults and can let go.

The merciful caregiver doesn't judge or apply conditions. She wants for others what she wants for herself. S/he is a loving advocate for residents, making sure they have what they need and deserve. Watch the exchange between a merciful caregiver and the patient, arms entwined when lifting; it can seem like a dance.

Our awareness of this even exchange is heightened when we consider the root of mercy, the word "merc." Merc is also the root of the words "commerce" and "merchant." Connected again with the basic image of exchange, these words suggest a value given and received between parties, as the seller and the buyer both gain.

Without a seller, there is no buyer. Without a caregiver there is no patient. Without showing mercy, one shall not receive it.

"What goes around comes around."

That's how Richard explained the turn of events. A CNA for thirteen years in Illinois, Richard Johnson had a bad day at work, one of his worst. "Imagine your worst day, then double it. That was my day."

A man who believes in the balance of the Universe, that what goes out through the window comes back through the door, Richard decided to review his life. He went on a personal hunting expedition, to find where and when he had not practiced the Golden Rule. Believing he had brought the day upon himself, as a reckoning for his own behavior, he looked honestly at his recent activities.

"I remembered there was a guy I owed $200 to, and I hadn't paid him back. That's what made everything go off the track." Holding ourselves accountable and recognizing the consequences of our actions is a powerful exercise. Seeing life as an exchange, a passing of good and bad energy, we can get a glimpse of our role in creation. Take a moment at the scene of the accident: did you cause it?

TODAY: *Look honestly at your actions.*

The late Representative Bob Harris, a Republican member of the Vermont House of Representatives, was a great proponent of a state lottery. He maintained Vermonters were crossing state borders to buy lottery tickets, and that was bad for the economy. After years of introducing legislation to create a lottery, Harris succeeded and Vermont joined the rest of the nation, establishing the state-sponsored lottery commission.

Not much later, Harris won the lottery. Honest. Few of us see such immediate fruits of our labors!

Recently I've heard of some efforts to increase world peace and end capital punishment. Every day at noon, worldwide, members of the Zen Peacemaker Order stop what they're doing and spend one minute in silent meditation for world peace. "Can you imagine what would happen if all the people in the world stopped what they were doing every day at noon and returned to the present moment?"

The Religious Organizing Against the Death Penalty Project was created to pull the religious community in the United States together to work against capital punishment. At 6 PM on days in the U.S. when an execution is taking place, members of the group ring their monastery bells to remind all of us that a life is being extinguished.

We are ultimately the recipients of every action we take. Let us practice our principles, knowing we will also benefit.

Caregivers resist the urge to take an eye for an eye, knowing full well that patients are often not responsible for their actions. Being hit, spit on, kicked or bitten, the merciful caregiver never strikes back. She says, "There, but for the grace of God, go I."

TODAY: *Create a loving world.*

Living in the center of the Universe, or the middle of nowhere, depending on your outlook, telephones are a true blessing. The airport is 90 minutes from my house and I can fly almost nowhere direct from Vermont. So, whenever possible, I suggest telephone meetings.

If we've spent some time together in person, phone meetings work well. I especially enjoy the energy of conference calls, when 15 or 20 nursing assistants from far and wide are all on the phone. We share news about projects and ideas, and sometimes listen to a guest expert conduct an in-service.

We once spent an intense hour discussing what happens when a caregiver is falsely accused of committing abuse. Story upon story was told of ruined careers and reputations. We were all deflated by the realization that an accused caregiver is presumed guilty by the entire system, and his or her life is never the same.

We closed the call with a few small business items, and I felt compelled to ask, "Would anyone like prayers?" I knew the callers and their great faith.

"I would, this is Teresa." "Me too, this is Wendy." "Me too, this is Tina." "Me too, this is Valerie."

Soon, every person on the call asked to be prayed for.

And why not? Giving all that they do, with so many pressures and responsibilities, they wanted all the help they could get. Talking has its limits; prayer does not.

TODAY: *Pray for each other.*

A director of nursing asked my advice on handling this situation: An alert female resident claimed an alert male resident grabbed her chin and kissed her, though she yelled, "Don't do that!" The male resident denied it happened.

Oh, if unwanted kisses were our worst problem, what a wonderful world this would be! In a closed environment such as a family, school or nursing home, we can lose perspective when facing such conflicts. We want to assure a safe environment and preserving residents' rights is essential. The U.S. Constitution promises the same protections. Does that mean leaders guarantee no unwanted events occur? That the neighbors' cats won't ruin my sandbox? That my wallet isn't stolen?

Realistic expectations are essential for caregivers, families, and residents. Men are men and women are women. We mustn't mislead families that we produce and direct daily fairy tales at the facility.

I bet Eve, our female resident, has complained other times in her life about unwanted attention. I also believe Adam has been charged before. I suggested staff talk with Eve to determine if she has unsettled or unresolved anger about previous unsolicited attention. Old age is not just a time of loss; it is also about reconciliation and coming to peace with our lives. By listening carefully, staff may help her heal an old wound and move on.

Could complaining be her way of getting attention? Is she unhappy in the facility?

As for Adam, it is wise to ask the CNAs if he is a joker, someone who pinches bottoms and pulls pranks. His CNAs know him almost as well as God does. Ask the family if he is a flirt. If so, watch where he hangs out. No point leaving newspaper on the wood stove. In such instances, keep perspective. Don't let fear of sanctions or lawsuits cause molehills to become mountains. Preserving rights and safety is a goal, not a guarantee. You can't control people. Life happens!

TODAY: *Keep perspective.*

We are creatures of habit. I can swear off chocolate, declaring it vice of the past. But somehow, months later, a Snickers bar proposes and I succumb. Mad at myself, I must also be merciful with the little girl inside.

It takes a lifetime to develop who we are and what we do. Odds are, the resident who asks for a midnight snack isn't starting a new tradition. Nor is the request for three sugars in his coffee anything novel.

Honoring these personal rituals is merciful and reasonable.

Today is my friend Rocky's birthday. Rocky has lived his whole life as a client of the mental health system, living in group homes on tiny government subsidies. His clothes have been hand-me-downs, rarely fitting properly. Pants have always been too long, needing to be cut. Shoes have been too big, necessitating extra pairs of socks.

At my insistence, my husband Thurmond agreed to measure Rocky for pants, which was a funny scene all by itself. Rocky and I then went shopping for pants that would fit without alteration and some new shoes.

At the shoe store, the salesman and I exchanged speechless moments as Rocky removed his socks. All 13 mismatched pairs. While he arrived in a size 10 1/2 boot, he was measured as needing a size 7. We ordered some 7 EEE shoes and went off to buy pants.

A week later I brought Rocky his new shoes. He had cut off the bottom of his new jeans, and stood in front of me with threads hanging from the uneven hems. "Rocky, what happened to your jeans?"

"I cut 'em," he told me, simply practicing his lifetime routine.

A few days later, Rocky traded his shoes for a pack of cigarettes (I was stunned he found another pair of 7EEE feet so easily!) telling me they were too small. He put his socks back on, all 26, and slipped comfortably into some size 10 1/2 boots.

Rocky is one of my best teachers. I pass on this lesson about the importance of respecting old habits. They're as comfortable as an old pair of jeans. Or boots.

TODAY: *Respect old habits.*

My grandmother Purcell once told me, "there is no value in comparison." I don't remember what provoked the statement, but I've always remembered the advice. Young mothers are especially susceptible to this habit, wondering why their babies aren't walking like the one-year-old next door.

As caregivers, our patients can get caught up in these Envy Olympics, worried that a roommate is more independent or better able to handle personal care. Caregivers themselves foolishly measure themselves against coworkers, wondering if they are as good at certain tasks.

Even if we decide we are better than another person at some skill or duty, how does this conclusion make the world a better place? To be merciful to others, the wise caregiver encourages acceptance all the way around. Our challenge is to see that we are doing our best at this moment in time, and appreciate what we have.

The genius Albert Einstein was considered a very late talker, not speaking until after he turned three. Instead of talking, he sang. When asked what he was singing, little Albert would say, "I'm making up songs for God."

Who would say that singing songs to God isn't as good as reciting the alphabet? Albert Einstein, like the rest of us, had his own path. May we all support each other, and the unique ways we express our gifts.

TODAY: *See your uniqueness.*

What Do I Feel?

What do I feel when I look into a resident's eyes?
I feel love.

What do I feel when I wash their faces?
I feel needed.

What do I feel when I talk to them?
I feel comfort.

What do I feel when I listen to what they have to say?
I feel understanding.

What do I feel when I see them smile?
I feel Jesus.

What do I feel when they tell me thank you?
I feel like I'm somebody.

—Loretha Morgan, CNA
Written to the residents of Carthage Health Care Center,
Carthage, Mississippi

TODAY: *Feel like somebody.*

I find it amazing how caregivers discover the quirky preferences of residents. "When she makes that noise, it means she's cold," Rhonda told me. "How do you know?" I asked in wonder. Rhonda looked at me like I didn't know how to read a stop sign. "I don't know, I just do."

Professional caregivers decipher noises, broken speech, no speech, hand signals, whatever clues are presented. "He only eats Alpha Bits, God forbid they stop making them!"

I watched a frustrated and impatient young mother at the airport, looking clueless about her toddler's tears. We began talking about raising children. "If we just listen to our kids, they'll let us know what they need," I said.

Mother and child safely on their plane, I sat and thought about what I had said. "It's true for everyone about everything! We just need to listen to people!" Sometimes, in the name of efficiency or expediency, we don't take time to listen. We imagine Mr. Brown is just like Mr. Green, and what works for one will work for the other.

Today, when you are with that hard-to-please or -understand resident, take an extra minute or two to listen. Listen with your eyes, ears, and hands. What does your resident need?

TODAY: *Listen for clues.*

Merci!

We might not know another word in French, but we brightly thank one another like citizens of Paris. Thanking one another we are engaging in a beautiful ritual that is practiced in every language and nation. Having received a kindness, we return the gesture with a word of thanks.

At the heart of *merci* is the old root word "merc," also the mother of mercy. *Merci* is the grateful response we give away, exchanging kindnesses with another.

When my son Elliot began working at McDonald's he came home with some interesting news: "Mom, McDonald's is just like you!" I couldn't imagine what he meant, as at that time, I hadn't eaten red meat in eight years.

"How am I like McDonald's?" I asked.

"Because they make us say 'thank you' all the time, too!"

Elliot was trained to end every communication with other employees by saying "thank you." "Order of fries and a small coffee, thank you." "Egg McMuffin and small orange juice, thank you."

To exchange another sign of mercy, why not switch to "*merci*" today? When someone says, "Why are you saying that?" have fun telling them you are sharing your gratitude and a bit of forgiveness, too.

TODAY: *Say merci.*

The Minute

With fearful eyes
She looks to me
"Will you please
just stay with me?"
Her face is wrinkled
Her hands are weak
Yet her eyes sparkled
With wisdom she could not speak.
I look at my watch
I am running late
But I sit a while
To ease her fearful state.
Finally I had to go
She smiled a toothless smile
And said, "Don't you know
I really love you so?"

—Stacey-Ann Morgan, CNA
Bridgeport, CT

TODAY: *Sit a while.*

A family member once suggested that putting a plastic bag over the head of a retarded neighbor child would be an act of mercy. "She can't be happy," he reasoned.

Assuming one's capacity to feel is linked to intelligence is just wrong. Regardless of our IQ, our emotions are intact and complete.

Working as a CNA in 1995, I spent some time in the special care unit at Maple Lane Nursing Home. One of my residents was a woman in her mid-seventies experiencing the turbocharged onset of Alzheimer's disease. Just one month earlier, she had been entertaining guests in her home. When we met, she could not understand what was happening to her, and cried sporadically all day long. "I'm so sorry, I don't know why I am crying, I just can't stop," she would tell me.

When I was a kid, I called women like Mrs. Daniels "classy." She was the wife of a corporate executive who had moved and set up a gracious home five times during her husband's career. A woman of style, she told me, "I have never let anyone see my cry, but I can't seem to control it anymore. I'm so sorry."

After each apology, I would touch her lightly and say, "Mrs. Daniels, you finally have time to cry. It is okay; you don't have to hold it back anymore." She would look at me with innocence and say, "How do you know? I think you may be right."

As Mrs. Daniels' mind continued to fade, her emotions took over. She no longer needed to bite her tongue, keep a stiff upper lip, keep her chin up or commit any other act of repression. She could feel her sorrow and anger and let it all out.

Caring for her during this highly charged time, the aides and nurses recognized the need for abundant mercy. After a lifetime of being the perfect wife and hostess, attentive to others, Mrs. Daniels now deserved the same quality of attention and comfort. It was our privilege.

TODAY: *Minister to emotions.*

I've never thought much about beards. My father shaved every morning with an electric razor. None of my friends' fathers had beards either. I think there were two or three professors or a scientist at church who had beards, but that was it.

Marrying a bearded man put beards in my consciousness for the first time. I learned that electric shavers aren't for everyone. I also learned that shaving could cause rashes and infections for men with sensitive skin. Have you thought about how much time is saved when shaving isn't part of the morning routine?

In the North Country, where I live, men with beards are abundant. Here, facial hair is more about the weather than fashion or appearance. When you're plowing snow or hunting deer, extra warmth is appreciated.

Being so beard-aware, I was stunned by how a facility I visited was treating its one resident with a beard: they kept trying to shave him! Staff talked about the dreaded chore with various levels of resolve. Phrases like "non-compliant" were used. Everyone agreed one aide was better than most at getting the gentleman shaved, though even she said some days it was like a rodeo.

"He tries to hit; he just won't stay still," she admitted.

"Why are you shaving him at all if he wants a beard?" I asked, making no attempt to hide my concern.

"The administrator says we have to," was the reply. I needed a moment of silence.

Today is my husband's birthday, and in his name, I write this request: let us honor the personal preferences of residents. Hair, whether it is on the face or the head, is not part of the building and grounds, subject to landscaping. May we ask no resident to get a haircut or beard trim or worse against his or her will. We are serving others, not controlling them.

TODAY: *Respect personal preferences.*

At age 48, I was confirmed as a Roman Catholic. I say it is the best decision I've made for the second half of my life.

Though some friends and family members didn't fully understand this step in my life, they were respectful when we talked about it. How I appreciated not being judged!

In my eyes, one of the most precious parts of the Catholic Mass is the reverence everyone exhibits when approaching the altar. I love reverence, and have been thinking about where else we see it expressed. New babies elicit a similar respectful behavior: we approach on tiptoe and hold them like paper-winged butterflies.

What if we were to greet all human beings with this same sense of awe? Can you imagine what it would be like to be sick and old, lying in a nursing home bed, and treated with such loving regard?

Another favorite part of the Mass is what we say just before receiving communion: "Lord, I am not worthy to receive you, but only say the word and I shall be healed." For the first two months I was a Catholic, I thought we were saying, "Only say the word and I shall be freed." When I discovered my error, I realized that by being healed, I was also freed. Freed of my pain, fear, sorrow, shame, and anger.

Merciful acts heal us and free us. The merciful touch of a loving caregiver can make loneliness disappear. In the Mass we ask the Lord to have mercy. Let us all be open to this request from others, and be a source of mercy wherever needed.

TODAY: *Be reverent and have mercy.*

Working with a know-it-all is no fun. No matter what you do, they have a better, quicker, easier, nicer way to do it. Though you are an adult, they somehow make you feel like an idiot. Or just angry. Or worse, an angry idiot.

Even more maddening is the moment you realize you are letting this annoying person make you feel stupid or mad. Yes, you let them control you; you surrender your mood and attitude to them. You might as well hand over your will and self-esteem and say, "Stomp here!" Regardless of how sure we are that the other person driving us nuts, the entire event is our choice.

You decide to be a doormat. What would happen if you just decided the know-it-all was just a silly critter, like a Dr. Seuss character? The Cat in the Hat can't affect you, and neither can this funny-face.

Dr. James Herriot, the veterinarian who wrote several wonderful books on his work and life in Wales, lived a happy life in large part because he didn't let anyone hurt him with scornful attitudes or words. He found a way to be amused by their harsh judgments or criticisms. Without his reaction, his accusers had no power.

When we practice mercy, we see how pointless it is to respond to the know-it-all with much more than a smile. For whatever reason, this poor soul needs to act this way. You, on the other hand, act the way you always do: mercifully.

TODAY: *Smile at the know-it-all.*

P.S. If you think you may be a know-it-all, feeling superior to coworkers, this could be a tip-off that you need to use your gifts in a larger fashion. Could it be you should be coaching, teaching or mentoring others? Going back to school? Applying for a promotion? Writing a book?

Liz had never worked anywhere but in a nursing home kitchen. She had been employed by many nursing homes, but always in the kitchen. For the past 18 years, she had managed kitchens. A professional, she liked to think she knew what made her residents happy, and she tried hard to use this knowledge.

Perhaps that is what made her so mad when the corporate dietary director, some 1,000 miles away, denied her request to buy mini birthday cakes for celebrating residents.

"People get sick of the same old thing. And no matter how we dress things up, our cakes all taste about the same. When you've lived here a while, the kitchen doesn't offer many surprises," Liz admitted.

So for birthdays, she liked to get a fancy single-serving cake from a local Italian bakery. "Their decoration is beautiful and we put a candle in it on the tray. I think it makes residents feel special."

But the cakes cost $2, and the budget-conscious dietician at headquarters rejected Liz's request to serve the Italian cakes to celebrants.

"I'm not a tough person to get along with," Liz said. "I'm a good employee and I treat the budget like it is my own money. But this decision made me mad. I make plenty of cakes, but I wanted something different. I was almost $8,000 under budget, and I knew I could buy those cakes. I appealed her decision."

Liz knew she might be labeled a troublemaker when she faxed in her carefully-worded appeal. "I saw it as a residents' rights issue. This could be their last birthday; why not make it a little special?" she wrote.

To her delight, the appeal was granted. "They paid attention and I convinced them. They know I put my residents first."

TODAY: *Advocate for birthday surprises.*

At age 13, when I blew out the candles of my birthday cake, I wished I would be 20. Somehow, I knew the rollercoaster ride of adolescence was ahead, and I just wanted to get on with the show.

Wanting to be a grown-up is a powerful urge that is gradually replaced by an equally powerful urge to slow down the biological clock. Where is that fountain of youth when we need it? Aging is regarded as a painful decline by the Western world, a time of diminished earning power:

> We deny it as long as possible, defeat it by compulsive productivity, or are distracted from it by activities and games. The Hindu model suggests a different approach: to use the very losses and diminishments of aging as our engine of spiritual growth.

With this Eastern approach we see aging as a time of a welcome detachment. Growing old is not a sad state marked by loss, but an opportunity to let go of duties, be liberated from material trappings and have time to do spiritual work.

My friend Dr. David Bryan refers to the final years of life as the fallow time. Comparing the stillness of old age with dormant farmland in the winter, David cautions us against thinking that this is a season of no activity. Underneath the snow plenty is happening—percolating, sifting and settling. Seniors can experience the same separating, working through and settling. Thinking that sitting residents are doing nothing can be a mistake, according to David Bryan. By briefly placing a hand on the arm or shoulder of a quiet resident, we let them know they aren't alone on their journey.

TODAY: *See aging as liberation.*

Occasionally we hear a nominee or candidate for a judge-ship being interrogated on his or her personal views of certain laws: "Would you be able to enforce laws you may oppose on religious or moral grounds?" I can't recall ever hearing someone answer no.

Working in a healthcare facility, we can find ourselves in the same boat, carrying out policies we don't support. When a new, budget-conscious administrator was hired, the staff was shocked by one of his early edicts: we will no longer use facility money to buy prizes for resident bingo games. Thinking he had discovered a way to save more than $300 ($6 a week), Mr. Humbug seemed genuinely surprised by the responses he got, not from the residents but from staff.

"How can you take away their one excitement for the week? They look forward to bingo more than anything else! Are you serious?"

Appealing to the senses of department heads, frontline staff pushed for a reversal of the policy. Some talked of taking up a collection to pay for bingo prizes.

To her credit, the fairly new director of nursing collected all the feedback and approached the administrator with tact and courtesy. In clear terms, she outlined what his decision had done to the facility's inside weather. Respectfully, she advised him he should immediately pull his decision and, at the same time, promise the staff he would not make this kind of mistake again.

"Making unilateral decisions with no staff or resident input on non-emergency issues is not your job. And it is no way to establish yourself here," she told him. Fortunately he listened, and today, while eyes roll when the bingo debacle is mentioned, a little laughter is also heard.

TODAY: *Don't mess with bingo!*

What does home mean? More specifically, what does it mean to be without a home?

Plenty of expressions are repeated daily in a nursing facility, but among the top ten is "I want to go home." Who wouldn't?

Thoughts of home are an instant source of calm and well-being. To be without a home suggests non-personhood, not belonging, uprootedness. Seeing oneself as homeless can cause feelings of disconnectedness, insecurity, and powerlessness.

What do we do when residents dwell on their dwelling? Listen.

Invite descriptions of the backyard, gardens, their favorite room. Did you have a real Christmas tree? Cut it down? Make your own decorations? Ask for a virtual tour of the property. Vivid sharing reminds residents that they still have access to the joy and comforts a home affords.

Perhaps you have moved from a favorite home yourself. For both of you, that old home is just a blink away: close your eyes and you're there.

Holding a resident discussion group on memories of home could be healing for participants. Stories about childhood homes complete with outhouses are wonderfully entertaining. How about inviting a classroom to visit, with students playing the part of reporters asking questions of Grandpersons? Mercy appears in many shapes and sizes. For those who are displaced, mercy is an empathetic ear.

TODAY: *Listen to memories.*

Social work students at Brigham Young University were asked to write what they learned working with their first clients. Rolf Halbfell, a student from Germany, wrote:

I've learned that you cannot make someone love you. All you can do is be someone who can be loved. The rest is up to them.

I've learned that no matter how much I care, some people just don't care back.

I've learned that it takes years to build up trust, and only seconds to destroy it.

I've learned that you shouldn't compare yourself to the best others can do.

I've learned that you can do something in an instant that will give you heartache for life.

I've learned that it's taking me a long time to become the person I want to be.

I've learned that you should always leave loved ones with loving words. It may be the last time you see them.

I've learned that you can keep going long after you can't.

I've learned that we are responsible for what we do, no matter how we feel.

I've learned that either you control your attitude or it controls you.

I've learned that heroes are the people who do what has to be done when it needs to be done, regardless of the consequences.

I've learned that money is a lousy way of keeping score.

I've learned that sometimes the people you expect to kick you when you're down will be the ones to help you get back up.

I've learned that sometimes when I'm angry I have the right to be angry, but that doesn't give me the right to be cruel.

I've learned that true friendship continues to grow, even over the longest distance. Same goes for true love.

I've learned that maturity has more to do with what types of experiences you've had and what you've learned from them and less to do with how many birthdays you've celebrated.

I've learned that you should never tell a child their dreams are unlikely or outlandish. Few things are more humiliating, and what a tragedy it would be if they believed it.

I've learned that no matter how good a friend is, they're going to hurt you every once in a while and you must forgive them for that.

I've learned that no matter how badly your heart is broken the world doesn't stop for your grief.

I've learned that we can't control our background and circumstances but we are responsible for who we become.

I've learned that we don't have to change friends if we understand that friends change.

I've learned that two people can look at the exact same thing and see something totally different.

I've learned that no matter how you try to protect your children, they will eventually get hurt and you will hurt in the process.

I've learned that even when you think you have no more to give, when a friend cries out to you, you will find the strength to help.

I've learned that credentials on the wall do not make you a decent human being.

I've learned that it's hard to determine where to draw the line between being nice and not hurting people's feelings and standing up for what you believe.

TODAY: *Write down what you've learned.*

Betty Jo had a "cling-on." Bill had been crazy about Betty Jo since her first day on the job. When she drew his name at the staff-resident Christmas party, his infatuation was total. Patients fall in love with their doctors, so a resident getting a crush on an aide shouldn't surprise us.

"Look what Betty Jo gave me for Christmas! Five pounds of cookies and a sweatshirt!" Bill beamed. Like a middle-schooler asking his girl to go steady, Bill gave Betty Jo his cross to wear.

"The thing is wooden and huge," Betty Jo told a coworker. "I admired it on Bill, and he insisted I take it. Now, every day he sees me, he has to check and see if I'm wearing the cross." A tiny woman, Betty Jo looks like a little girl playing dress up, pretending she's a nun.

"Some days I forget to put it on, or I just don't feel like having it clang around my neck," she admitted. "But the minute I see Bill, I realize what a mistake I've made. He won't leave me alone."

By confiding in another employee, Betty Jo was able to unload some of her confusion without hurting Bill. They discussed her options, and decided she would tell Bill that on his birthday, a month away, he would be getting the cross back as a special gift from her. Her coworker also promised to give Bill some extra attention, so he might begin to spread his affection a little further.

TODAY: *Deal mercifully with crushes.*

We had Julia's first care plan meeting at Union House and she enjoyed herself. Sitting next to each other, we held hands and listened to the staff's report on her condition and adjustment to her new home.

Talking about interests and activities, I shared some stories of Julia's great talent as a craftswoman. "My piano bench has a lovely hooked rug on it that Julia made me. We also have some pillow cases she embroidered with big colorful roses." Thinking I was giving Julia cause for great pride, I continued.

"At Project Independence, Julia would work on 500-piece puzzles, do coloring and make jewelry with beads. She can do anything with her hands!"

After the meeting, Julia and I went to sit together for a while. Over coffee and juice, she had a sad face. "I'm sorry I don't do crafts anymore; I just don't," she said apologetically.

I immediately recognized the pain I had inadvertently caused. Julia misunderstood my reminiscence, and thought I was disappointed in her for no longer doing handwork. She again apologized, somewhat wistfully. After stumbling a few minutes, I seized on the concept of retirement, and announced that now that she had retired, she didn't have to do anything she didn't want to do. She seemed to relax at the thought, and was able to stop apologizing.

I left feeling I had hurt her, and also knowing I had learned a valuable lesson. I promised myself that I would be more careful talking about the old days with Julia. Who she is and what she is doing this very moment is absolutely perfect.

TODAY: *Be sensitive to misunderstandings.*

I am quite certain humans have been trying to prolong life since first encountering death. Struggling to live forever is as old as the hills, and as advanced as the Internet.

We may have the machinery to keep people alive, but is that what any of us actually want? No one asked—they just invented. Technology has raced ahead of our ability to define what a quality life looks like.

The late Henri J. M. Nouwen wrote, "Technology is so far ahead of human relations! There is such a need for new ways for people to be together, to solve conflicts, to work for peace."

Grace, a social worker, said she was pressured by facility nurses to get Do No Resuscitate (DNR) orders from families. "The nurses don't like to do resuscitation," Grace said. Making this gigantic issue the social worker's alone is not appropriate. Why not create a booklet to give to family members at admission? Can a statement be added to the admissions agreement so the matter is dealt with early and up-front, as part of the routine paperwork?

When I admitted Julia into Union House, shuffled in with all the papers was the DNR form. I was also asked if Julia was to have flu shots, if she'd had a pneumonia vaccine, and if the application for Medicaid had been submitted. Everything felt routine and was handled on the spot.

Regardless of how the facility solicits family DNR preferences, one truth remains: nurses are paid to resuscitate patients, whether they want to or not. Most patients are more frightened of death than resuscitation. Unless clear directions are given, resuscitation is required.

TODAY: *Be clear about DNRs.*

(Reprinted from *The Road to Daybreak, A Spiritual Journey* by Henri J. M. Nouwen. New York, Doubleday Books. Copyright © 1988 p. 183)

Despite the dramatic high-tech advances in medicine, the lowly aspirin is still considered one of the best defenses against a second heart attack or stroke. Sometimes old-fashioned remedies are unbeatable.

In 1837, Charles Hendee published *The Family Nurse, or Companion of the American Frugal Housewife* by Mrs. Child. The book's first sentence stresses it "is by no means intended to supersede the advice of a physician." Yet it is full of advice physicians would be wise to pass along:

> A real good nurse must have a tender conscience, as well as a feeling heart. She must realize that the slightest deviation from the truth, even to screen herself from blame, is not only a violation of the trust reposed in her, but is a sin against God.

> When her patience is severely taxed by unreasonable caprices, she must remember how sickness weakens the mind, and try to apply the golden rule.

> When infants are fretful, she must beware of the temptation to administer opiates. To endanger the health, or dim the intellect of a human being, for the sake of temporary convenience, is a fearful responsibility.

Wise advice for those who care for fretful elders, as well.

Not all homespun treatments are still in vogue. I am a bit wary of Mrs. Child's cure for hysteric fainting fits: "The odor of burning feathers, horn or leather is good."

You work with a wise, wise group of men and women, professional caregivers who have learned over decades successful ways of handling myriad challenges. I have long believed there isn't a nursing home problem of any significance that nursing assistants aren't able to solve. When facing a tough situation, find your longest-serving associates and pick their brains.

TODAY: *Look for proven remedies.*

Out of curiosity, I like to ask alert nursing home residents about their preferences.

"Do you like being awakened in the morning, or would you rather sleep in and wake up naturally?"

So far, only a handful of women have told me they like being wakened. I'm not surprised. When one of our three dogs wakes me up with either a bark or a lick, I rarely grin. I love my trio, but I also like to finish my dreams before I open my eyes. If they were to make me get up and be fully dressed at the breakfast table in 8 or 10 minutes, I would be very grouchy!

Let's add one more factor to this scenario: retirement. Not having to get up to catch a bus or carpool or punch a time clock, why would anyone who is frail and infirm want to be awakened from a sound sleep?

When I ask nursing home staff why residents are propped up in dining rooms across the country at 7 AM, most answers reference regulations or facility convenience. I have never had one caregiver tell me they wake residents for the residents' sake.

Hmmm. What would the merciful action be? How would we like our mornings to look? I would like to use the toilet and get back into bed, have a hot drink, coffee on some days, tea on others, and two pieces of toast. If, God willing, I still can read, I would love a newspaper and my devotionals. Later, I would appreciate some help getting dressed, and you can forget the bra, thank you very much.

What would you like? What would your residents like? Isn't it time to deliver what the customer ordered?

TODAY: *Ask customers to choose.*

We are spoiled in the U.S., but don't tell us that when we're complaining.

Remember the routine about starving kids in Africa who would love your untouched plateful of liver and onions? Somehow their existence only made us mad. "Send it to 'em!" we thought, but if we were smart, didn't say.

Assisted living facilities are the bed of choice these days, and the reasons are obvious: private bedroom, private bath and often a kitchenette, the design acknowledges our individual desires for privacy and independence. Though I have yet to meet a single assisted living resident who prefers to cook instead of enjoy the prepared meals that are provided, I know teeny kitchens are a big selling point. A kitchen symbolizes freedom. Though kitchen sinks and stoves are often used to store yarn or magazines, nevertheless they are there for all to see.

Old nursing homes offer none of these feel-good features. Three or four residents in one bedroom is still a fairly common arrangement. That generally means six people are sharing a bathroom. Sounds like our childhoods!

While most of the world shares bathrooms that are less sophisticated than a nursing home bathroom, like the kids in Africa, this doesn't make the lack of privacy feel any more acceptable. Telling residents who are unhappy living in a "gang room" that elders in Third World countries share a bed with three grandchildren isn't helpful.

Feeling stacked like airplanes over O'Hare airport is real to the resident, and when they tell you about this discomfort, they are looking for relief. Staff at a Midwest facility I worked with decided to focus on offering more activities, encouraging residents to only use their rooms for sleeping. "We adopted the attitude that our facility was like summer camp, and people only go to their beds to sleep."

TODAY: *Offer relief to the crowded.*

Hearing an 88-year-old woman argue with her sixty-some-year-old daughter about the moral character of a drag queen is a unique experience.

Gary is a nursing assistant and a professional female impersonator. At work, while he is in uniform, his long blond hair and sculpted fingernails remain part of his look. An extraordinarily optimistic and competent CNA, Gary is universally respected by coworkers and residents alike.

Living and working within a small, one-story facility, relationships are close. When you are 88-year-old Mabel and need to get to the bathroom in the middle of the night, what the caring person who answers the call light does as his weekend job isn't too important. What matters is that Gary is reliable and merciful. Mabel loves Gary and she told her daughter so.

Without experiencing any of this intimate bonding, the sixty-something children of residents deal only with surface appearances: "Mother, how can you tolerate being around him?"

I am heartened by this story, as it confirms an ancient truth: when we know one another, we cannot hate. Conventional thinking suggests that old dogs can't be taught new tricks, and women in their late eighties are stereotyped as stuck in their ways. Mabel dispels this myth, and gives fresh proof of the glorious possibilities brought on by proximity. Intolerance doesn't have to rule when friendship has a chance.

TODAY: *Know the heart first.*

When Julia started to fall at the facility, I realized she wasn't wearing her own glasses. "She didn't arrive with glasses," the staff said, noting this was a most common occurrence. "That's why she keeps showing up with Jean's glasses on."

In the confusion of a move, such oversights can be expected. Hearing aids, walkers, canes and other prosthetic devices are left behind, misplaced or just plain disappear. When a guardian or distant relative is handling the transfer, the chances for a mishap multiply.

I was so grateful that Union House staff talked to me about the falls before they made any extreme decisions. I've heard about medication-happy facilities where anti-vertigo drugs are prescribed. Residents who fall can also be discouraged from roaming freely, sometimes confined to tilted-back chairs that they can't get out of alone.

As Julia's guardian, it is my responsibility to follow up with the director of nursing, to make sure an eye appointment has been scheduled. With 50 other residents to watch over, Brooke isn't infallible. Rather than assume the facility has everything under control, I will maintain my sense of duty in Julia's life and stay on top of her falling and need for glasses.

TODAY: *Look for simple solutions.*

Marguerite did not have a supportive family. Her sons were elderly themselves, and showed little interest in their mother's phone calls. A nursing home resident for nearly 10 years, Marguerite had made few friends in the facility.

Her aide, Therese, was her best friend. When other aides got exasperated with Marguerite's moods or demands, Therese kept her even temperament and merciful touch. Without judgment or impatience, Therese handled Marguerite with loving diplomacy.

"I want to talk to my son in California!" Marguerite began yelling the night before. When Therese came on duty, Marguerite was wound tight. "Just before my break, I will dial the number for you," Therese promised.

Because the phone nearest Marguerite's room was a wall phone, she couldn't reach it from her wheelchair. She insisted on using this phone, probably because that meant someone had to stay with her to hang up. Therese dialed and stood beside Marguerite during the call. True to form, Marguerite and her son were fighting about the past just a few minutes into the call. Suddenly, Marguerite shouted, "Well, someone who does care about me is going to hang up on you now!" and handed the phone to Therese. With great satisfaction, Marguerite watched Therese place the phone in its cradle.

Remembering to invest no strong feelings in the whole encounter, Therese protected herself from getting sucked into taking sides in this dysfunctional family. She kept her focus on meeting Marguerite's needs with practicality and mercy. Can you think of a resident who could benefit from this light touch?

TODAY: *Stand by your residents.*

My father recites the promise the U.S. Marine Corps made to enlistees in World War II: three hots and a cot. Stationed on Iwo Jima, he learned the Marines couldn't always keep that promise of providing breakfast, lunch, dinner and a bed.

Nursing homes make similar promises to residents, referencing the minimum licensing standards outlined by the federal government. During the annual state surveys, inspectors determine if the facility is meeting these minimum standards of care.

But is achieving a passing score at providing the minimum truly a level of service worth bragging about? Could providers make a more complete promise to residents?

When my friends Gary and Alicia Marcotte owned Maple Lane Nursing Home, their personal definition of quality care far exceeded any national or state minimums. Residents and family members confirm the superiority of the Marcotte promise with their memories.

Michael Gruteke, who has lived in many nursing homes and facilities in several states, fondly recalls Gary's "above and beyond" kindnesses:

> My grandfather had been a ham radio operator and I picked up his interest. I studied for the radio operator's license and wanted to set up my own base in the nursing home. Gary made it happen; he even got the antenna on the roof for me.

Today, Mike lives independently, with one whole wall of his apartment dedicated to his ham station. Since leaving Maple Lane, he has been licensed to transmit at more advanced levels, is an officer in the state ham radio club and travels to national conventions of the Handi Hams. "I will never forget what Gary did for me," Mike says.

TODAY: *Maintain your own high standards.*

As children, we all have ideas or fantasies about what life will be like when we are grown up. I knew I wanted to help people, and I also knew I loved to write. As a little boy my brother Will would find a subject that fascinated him and devour whatever information he could find on it. Today, he heads up a research division in a national corporation. My other brother, Tim, always said he would be an FBI agent. He is a federal judge, so that seems pretty close.

Imagining our work and family lives is pretty common. But who would think that someday they would become a central ritual in another person's life?

Donna didn't talk much about her work as a nursing assistant in a large, urban facility. Dependable and respected, she had been taking care of people since her children graduated from high school. Now in her late fifties, she was reflecting on her life and its meaning.

"I have been wondering if I have amounted to anything," she said candidly at an informal gathering of other CNAs. "You look back and think, 'did it mean anything?'" Other voices chimed in, and the discussion turned to sharing examples of individual residents who had become dependent on their aides.

"I just got to thinking about one of my residents, Pearl," Donna said. "Every day she says she can't start her day without a kiss from me. Maybe it sounds funny, but she means it. I make sure I am in her room first thing each morning so she gets her kiss. Pearl always says the same thing, 'Now I can have a good day.'"

Take a moment to review your patterns of care at work, particularly related to rituals. What simple acts of kindness and mercy do you practice regularly, boosting the morale or well-being of another? Notice the rituals you are part of, and treasure this truth.

TODAY: *Enjoy rituals of care.*

Most nursing homes house residents who are veterans of military service, some of whom have seen active combat. Activities directors often will plan events around the Memorial Day holiday, inviting members of the local VFW or American Legion to come to the facility and conduct a flag-raising ceremony that salutes residents who once were in uniform.

To other departments, planning such celebrations can look like an easy job. Few people realize the number of phone calls, dead ends, new contacts and arrangements the activities department has to pursue. Communities have a couple of color guards available, and their services are in great demand.

My friend Sandy DeForge, one of the finest activities directors I've ever met, is known for her persistence in tracking down the right people to lead programs. A professional, she recognizes the value of providing visual stimulation from the outside to residents.

I remember watching the staff's surprise when, following a Memorial Day mini-parade, a withdrawn male resident began an animated talk about his years stationed overseas in the U.S. Army, fighting the Nazis. Until that moment, he had said nothing about this emotional time in his life. CNAs were delighted to hear him open up, and called it the turning point: "We have gotten to know him because of the little parade."

Offering a change of scenery or creating a special event for residents can call forth stories not heard before. In some cases, the atmosphere and timing is so perfect that a painful memory may be spoken for the first time ever. The simple visit of a serviceman in uniform can trigger the telling of tragic tales. Be prepared to hear wartime memories of family members who enlisted and never came home. Help your residents heal.

TODAY: *Prepare to hear painful memories.*

June: Blessed are the pure in heart for they shall see God

For the pure of heart, as the poet Shelley wrote, virtue is its own reward. Serving—not helping—the pure of heart consider caring an honor, an opportunity to love as God loves.

This Beatitude promises that when one's inside world is right, s/he will see beauty in the outside world. When others may be blind, the pure of heart see God in the faces and interactions of each new day. The pure see with pure eyes, seeing all things as pure. Such spiritual purity is a requirement for true caring, since a pure, clean heart has the greatest influence on behavior.

Caregivers who are pure of heart approach their work and their clients without needing a social reference. It matters not if a resident is a former janitor or a retired lawyer. Each individual is accepted with equal and unwavering reverence, welcomed like a blooming rose in the garden, worthy of wholehearted attention. This level of intimacy is not one of false closeness, where light pleasantries or nicknames imitate real relationship. Instead, theirs is a meeting of the souls.

The pure heart represents the whole personality, the center of the inner life, the source of thought, understanding, will and decision. The pure life demands a full transformation at these deepest levels. Like pure linen, gold or glass, the pure heart is clean and clear, untainted by alloys.

Such people don't focus on the physical side of life, as their purity is drawn from inside. Strong and clear-headed, they fear nothing, free from negativity and phoniness. External pressures don't have power over them. But don't be fooled! Simply presenting an outward appearance of purity, which almost anyone can accomplish, will not bring strength or the gift of seeing beauty. Only a private and personal purity delivers.

Impure people make everything dirty. Listening to their off-color jokes or derogatory remarks we feel dirty. To preserve our own well-being, we must keep our distance.

All communities need the pure of heart if genuine harmony is to be experienced. The law-abiding and moral are needed, but without the pure of heart, the innermost beauty of individuals is neither revealed nor seen. Blessed be the pure of heart.

"I was only 18 when I first started working in a nursing home," Carolyn remembered. "Luckily, I had Elsie to take care of."

A member of Beverly Healthcare's National CNA Leadership Council, Carolyn Barge, a CNA at Gray's Harbor Nursing Center in Aberdeen, WA, is a consummate observer of residents.

Elsie was petite, and paralyzed on the left side by a stroke. "She was always so uplifting and a great source of comfort and encouragement. She never complained about herself, and I loved her dearly," Carolyn said.

"When she fell ill and died, I cried so hard. There are times when I get busy and stressed, and I think of her, and I can still hear her words of encouragement. It helps me to get through those times."

Wise caregivers know when they need a booster shot, and where to get it. As a career nursing assistant, Carolyn learned early on that she could look to others, particularly residents, for inspiration and hope. Rather than seeing Elsie as broken, Carolyn looked and listened clearly, and found a great source of strength and support. Long after Elsie died, Carolyn still summons these memories.

Outsiders tend to misunderstand the nature of your work. Far from a one-way street, quality caregiving is an exchange of spirit. Being open to the contributions of others, the mature caregiver receives as she gives, seeing God in all.

TODAY: *Accept blessings from residents.*

If you know anyone looking for a wonderful dissertation topic, suggest this: research the phenomenon of babies born in the late 1920s or early 1930s named Millie.

Let's talk about The Millies. To date, I've met three, and they are all outstanding caregivers working well beyond traditional retirement dates. Millie Aldrich is in Mishawaka, IN, in her early seventies. You met her on February 20.

Millie Heath has a summer camp on my road. She is in her 80s, grandmothered into Vermont's licensure of practical nurses since she was nursing before the profession was regulated. She describes working as a private duty home health nurse as "driving to the homes of old ladies and taking care of them."

Millie Jennings is outside of Cleveland, Ohio, at a nursing home owned and operated by the Little Sisters of the Poor. An active nursing assistant, Millie whispered to me at our first meeting, "Don't tell anyone I'm 75; they'll want to make me retire."

Old enough to be nursing home residents, The Millies are age-defying wonders. Sisters at Millie Jennings' facility like to tell the story of the massive snowstorm where no employees made it to work. Well, none but Millie. "We saw her coming down the hall in her galoshes, a little after 3PM," recalls Sister Lorraine. "All she was saying was 'I'm sorry for being a little late.'"

Look around for these pillars in your facility: men and women who stay young and vital caring for others. Do you have any Millies? Or Willies? While they could be known by any name, their performances will reveal their pure hearts.

My book of baby names lists the meaning of Millie as The Comforter. I'm not surprised.

TODAY: *Praise the Millies.*

Mr. Powell has faithfully visited his wife's bedside daily since she entered the nursing home seven years ago. Diagnosed with Parkinson's disease, some days Mrs. Powell doesn't seem to know her husband of 53 years. Still, he arrives at noon to make sure his wife eats a hot meal.

"I know the girls are busy, so I figure I can help feed my wife before her food cools. They told me the government says it is illegal for volunteers to help feed anyone but their own family, so only I can help her." (Good old government, protecting nursing homes from the attentions of others! Have to wonder how so many folks survive at home, being fed by friends and neighbors without government protection.)

That particular Wednesday, Mrs. Powell wanted nothing to do with her husband. He tried for more than half an hour, but she refused the meal. Marybeth, the activities director, recognized his exasperation.

"How about you, Mr. Powell? Have you had any lunch today?" she asked the elderly gentleman as he left the dining room. He answered no, and relayed his frustration, "I just had to get out of there."

"We had a wonderful catered banquet for our veteran employees today, and there are lots of delicious leftovers in the break room," Marybeth volunteered. "Let me heat you up a plate and we'll sit and talk."

Minutes later, Marybeth and Mr. Powell were tucked into a quiet corner, chatting. Marybeth made sure this loving husband had a hot meal.

TODAY: *Serve families.*

Nationally there is a call to place hidden cameras, called Granny Cams, throughout nursing homes. "Put cameras in every room," it is said, "including the break room, hallways, and dining room, and there will be changes made."

My son Elliot is now a grown man. In all the years I enjoyed raising him, I never once witnessed him improving as a person when I lost faith in him. In fact, only when I encouraged him to do the right thing and expressed trust in his judgment did he rise to the occasion. My mothering taught me that people grow into our expectations of them.

External controls on human behavior may feel like the solution, but in my short 48 years on the planet, I have come to believe strongly that we cannot make others be better people. I regard the Granny Cams as insulting to staff and residents.

Internal personal controls, such a pure heart and mind, are the only certain guarantees of quality care. I believe what is needed is not more surveillance and less trust, but more community support and resources.

As a society, we must recognize and appreciate our caregivers. All human service providers deserve to be paid a living wage and given more education, recognition and standing. America must come to see those who take care of our parents and grandparents as worthy of respect.

Why work as a nursing assistant these days when the media and public so clearly mistrust you, to the point that 24-hour surveillance cameras are considered legitimate ways to improve care? Technology is not always the answer. Nor is rage.

As long as most Americans opt not to save for their old age, leaving government with the nursing home bill, nursing assistants will continue to be underpaid and mistrusted. Government pays as little as possible, and we get what we pay for: too few skilled staff.

Finding blame is an easy game. Taking responsibility isn't. Nursing homes run a bare-bones operation. What do we expect for $100 a day? That's what a hotel charges, with no nurse aide included.

Nursing homes need our help. If we had 100 volunteers at every facility, helping in a hundred different ways, all of our loved ones living in nursing homes would be happier.

TODAY: *Solicit some volunteers.*

Today's question: "What's age got to do with it?" focuses on the qualifications of a good caregiver. Does experience make all the difference?

Canadian home care worker Laurie Sandmaier answers from personal experience, reflecting on her aunt's home care team:

> I've had the privilege of meeting some of these happy, cheerful, caring and knowledgeable ladies. A few have been young but enthusiastic, with a goal to improve Aunt Chris's quality of life. Some have been more mature, bringing their life experiences into the equation, and they and Aunt Chris have a great time reminiscing.
>
> Whether these workers are fresh out of school, perhaps gaining experience on their way to becoming nurses, or skilled caregivers still doing this after 20 years because of their commitment to make a difference, Aunt Chris has truly benefited from their service.

The temptation to judge a coworker's qualifications and abilities are great. How many times have you heard, "I can spot a bad aide at 100 feet!" "I can tell if they aren't going to make it!" In response to these generalizations, I always suggest the critic look carefully at the people who work at her facility. Do they all look the same?

More than age, body type or nationality, the secret to becoming a successful caregiver lies in the purity of the heart. We each can think of innocent and tender new aides whose loving instincts made up for whatever they lacked in experience. And The Millies of June 2 are clear proof that caregivers are never too old. Age has nothing to do with it. Look to the heart for evidence.

TODAY: *Beware of age discrimination.*

Author Rachel Naomi Remen, MD writes:

> Serving is different from helping. Helping is based on inequality; it is not a relationship between equals. When you help you use your own strength to help those of lesser strength. If I'm attentive to what's going on inside of me when I'm helping, I find that I'm always helping someone who's not as strong as I am, who is needier than I am. People feel this inequality. When we help we may inadvertently take away from people more than we could ever give them; we may diminish their self-esteem, their sense of worth, integrity and wholeness.

Appreciating the distinction between helping and serving is a delicate matter. In the old days, helpers took extraordinary liberties in the name of "my client's best interests." Looking at our nation's nursing homes in the 1970s and 80s, restraints were popular "best practices," considered the best way to assure resident safety. Under the broad category of "helping," some fairly cruel treatments were sanctioned. Dr. Reman continues:

> Service is the relationship between equals. . .We can only serve that to which we are profoundly connected, that which we are willing to touch. This is Mother Teresa's basic message: We serve life not because it is broken, but because it is holy. . .Our service serves us as well as others. That which uses us strengthens us. Over time, fixing and helping are draining, depleting. Over time we burn out. Service is renewing. When we serve, our work itself will sustain us.

Serving rather than helping offers caregivers great freedom. Any sense of burden or exhaustion is removed. The resident is seen as a whole person needing assistance, not a broken being needing repair. With both parties regarded as whole and complete, the relationship between caregiver and cared-for can be full of fun and joy.

TODAY: *Serve.*

The Omnibus Reconciliation Act of 1987, OBRA '87, is still considered America's most sweeping federal reform of the nursing home industry. The law mandated such basics as 75 hours of nurse aide training and the proper use of restraints.

Long before OBRA-based surveys, when caring for residents good caregivers have consulted their pure hearts when determining the right thing to do.

Based on the OBRA, the Code of Federal Regulations, CFR, includes federal tags (F-tags) that are used to cite a facility's deficiencies during the annual survey. Can you translate these F-tags into your personal, internal language? Rewrite these rules into words that speak to the spirit, yours and your residents'.

F240: Quality of Life. A facility must care for its residents in a manner and in an environment that promotes maintenance or enhancement of each resident's quality of life.

F241: Dignity. The facility must promote care for residents in a manner and in an environment that maintains or enhances each resident's dignity and respect in full recognition of his or her individuality.

F242: Self determination and participation. The resident has the right to 1. choose activities, schedules, and health care consistent with his or her interests, assessments, and plans of care; 2. interact with members of the community both inside and outside the facility; and 3. make choices about aspects of his or her life in the facility that are significant to the resident.

F245: Participation in other activities. A resident has a right to participate in social, religious and community activities that do not interfere with the rights of other residents in the facility.

F246: Accommodation of needs. A resident has a right to reside and receive services in the facility with reasonable accommodations of individual needs and preferences, except when the health or safety of the individual or other residents would be endangered.

TODAY: *Strive for quality. (F240)*
Respect uniqueness. (F241)
Encourage and follow resident preferences. (F242)
Promote participation. (F245)
Serve special needs. (F246)

Yesterday, I received a message to pray for the life of Tamika Jackson, the five-year-old daughter of an Alabama nursing assistant. "She is very sick," my friend wrote.

Many of us find great comfort and solace in prayer. We also find results. Hearing of a terrible tragedy, we often feel helpless; the pain and loss are so great. Unable to magically fix what's broken, we say, "All I can do is pray, so that's what I'll do, I'll just pray about it."

Prayers offered with such a defeatist attitude make me smile. What makes us think prayer is such a discount offering to people in trouble? Do we think our human actions are superior to prayer?

I tease my mother, a Unitarian Universalist, and ask her to send me good UU vibes when I need them. However we describe intense thoughts we have for others, we know from personal experience they can make a difference.

In my own prayer life, I had a powerful revelation. I often pray to be made a better person with a purer heart. I ask for less ego and more compassion. "Be that person," said the voice from within. "Be who you pray you will become."

So what does a woman with a purer heart look like? I must be her. So what does the person you want to be look like? Be that person.

TODAY: *Be what you pray for.*

"Nobody talks to anyone! None of the guys from my shop even goes anymore; it's no fun." My friend was describing his company's annual party, and explaining why he and his wife decided not to go. Though the whole meal is free, in a beautiful restaurant, the awkward strain is more than they can bear.

We all know exactly what he described. Emotional discomfort, be it at a party, visiting someone's house, an office or a healthcare facility, is the feeling that makes you want to keep your coat on.

Many of us have had to end marriages because of extreme experiences of emotional discomfort. I always thought I had chronic constipation the entire ten years of my first marriage. Imagine my surprise when I moved into my own place and found all my personal plumbing worked perfectly! My body had been trying to tell me I wasn't dealing with the emotional discomfort.

Deciding if we belong where we are is a tough challenge. Many of us have reactions that aren't based on facts, but on habit. Some folks are known for running, so their tendency is to quit. Others are so afraid of change they tend to stay even when the suffering is unbearable.

Taking a step back and looking at a situation without emotional discomfort is what's needed. What is good about the place? Does it outweigh the bad? After all, we know that everywhere we go the ideal will elude us.

The writer Jean Toomer described seeing ordinary men living lives that "did not measure up to the worth and dignity of human lives and his longing for the unnamed things that did."

To a degree, we all long for purer, higher forms of life. What would it be like to live and work with people who valued life above all else? Can you manage the emotional discomfort in your life, and strive for a purer way of being?

TODAY: *Manage emotional discomfort.*

I was bouncing along in that wonderful trance induced by train travel when some words imbedded in the train window caught my eye: "Test proof window."

What test? What did that mean? How do you test a window? I thought about it. They must try to break it or cloud it up or make it crack or chip.

Am I a test proof woman? Every day I face the world and risk not only being broken but breaking someone else. Can I design a daily test or set of questions to ask myself, to see if I am continuing to be the pure heart I so desire?

Galatians 6:4 says:

> Each man should examine his own conduct for himself; then he can measure his own achievement by comparing himself with himself and not with anyone else. For everyone has his own proper burden to bear.

Think about customizing a simple test, maybe five questions you can tick off on your fingers, which will help you live the life you desire. Mine:

1. Did I take time for meditation and prayer?
2. Did I appreciate beauty?
3. Did I remember to laugh and say thank you?
4. Did I eat, sleep and exercise well?
5. Did I care for others?

TODAY: *Create your test.*

We sat in St. Anne's Cathedral on Donegal Street in Belfast, Northern Ireland, attending the city's first inter-faith celebration of peace. What an afternoon—one I will never forget!

Representatives from seven faiths participated in the program, which included song, music, dance, prayer and chanting. I doubt I will ever see a more beautiful, more pure-of-heart young dancer than Gayatri Bhatt, performing the Hindu Bharat Natyam dance. Of her performance, the program stated: "To watch the dancing and hear the chanting brings peace to the heart, mind and body."

Readings were also presented from the Hebrew scriptures on the Jewish view on peace, from the Holy Qu'ran on Luqman's instructions to his son on how to live his life, and from the holy texts of the Christian and Sikh traditions. Zhenia Mahdi-Nau sang the Persian chant "O Thou Kind Lord! Thou hast created all humanity from the same stock."

Seeing people from many nations and faiths celebrating the gift that is life lifted everyone present. We became one pure heart. The Buddhist meditation, sharing loving-kindness with one another, spoke what each of us felt.

Please accept my gift to you of the meditation and share it with others: "I send love and compassion to myself. I send love and compassion to all those around me. I send love and compassion to the whole country. I send love and compassion to the entire world. I wish no suffering, pain, anxiety or hurt for anyone."

Praying this ever-widening circle, until we encompass the earth with our love, is a powerful practice. After praying for all, look at how your thoughts and actions travel, and the consequences. In the privacy of your own heart and mind, you can change the world.

TODAY: *Become one pure heart.*

In 1997 I began a three-year adventure working with the world's largest provider of nursing home care, Beverly Healthcare. My mission was to create a new company awareness for the contributions and value of nursing assistants. Among my most wonderful assignments was to organize and staff the new National CNA Leadership Council.

In May of 2000, the Council hosted a banquet for corporate office leadership. For the first time, CNAs sat with home office associates and discussed their common goals. Everyone present regarded the evening as a rare and worthwhile opportunity.

When I first learned that Beverly was headquartered in Fort Smith, Arkansas, I scratched my head. Nothing flies direct to Fort Smith! Later, I learned some of the company's founders were from this area. I also learned of the presence of St. Scholastica Monastery, a Benedictine convent in town. The National Council members stayed at the convent and enjoyed the beautiful grounds. We also had the privilege of meeting Sister Cabrini Schmitz, who directs the Order's retreat center. Sister Cabrini led us all in a blessing at the Council banquet, and this is, in part, what she said:

> Thank you God for planting the seed of your own tenderness, compassion, loving and caring within the hearts of these men and women. May all see their work in Beverly facilities as continuing in your Son's own touching, healing ministry with each precious person they serve. And dear God, give all of us the gift of reverence; let us hold each person we meet as a sacred gift, no matter the wrapping. Teach us to love as you love.

TODAY: *Hold each person as a sacred gift.*

Some break room entertainment:

Call all the troops together for a science lesson. Take a glass or coffee cup, fill it with water to the top and then a little more. Make sure everyone notices that you actually fill the glass past the brim and it doesn't spill. Doing your best impression of Mr. Wizard, look at your students and say, "See? Water molecules attract each other quite closely. The surface tension keeps the water from spilling over the edge or pulling away."

So, Brainy One, what's your point?

"Now that we all understand surface tension and how it pulls everything together against the odds, I want to know this: what is the surface tension of our staff? What pulls us together?"

Healthy facilities rally around the residents. Regardless of personal problems or the crisis of the day, good caregivers remember their overriding purpose: to provide a loving and comfortable home for older men and women in need of care. On tough days, gossip or short-staffing can pull us off track, and we lose sight of what's important, what called us to this vocation. On such days, go to the BAR to escape: that's Breathe And Relax. Collect yourself and others; let the spirit of good care pull you all together again.

TODAY: *Pull together.*

Dog owners know one of the many joys our pets provide is the excited greeting. No matter how recently I've seen my little Maltese, when he comes back into the room he acts like we've been separated for a month. His whole body wags with love.

All creatures have special stages and unique behaviors. Watching our puppies and babies go through phases is especially delightful; each new skill or act is cause for a picture and celebration. And while we continue to enter new stages as we age, finding a reason to be joyous is sometimes hard. Ask family members of Alzheimer's patients, who must stand by, powerless, as their loved one loses another function or memory.

Extraordinary caregivers bring a gentle sense of acceptance and ease to whatever the day brings. Above all else, they treasure the precious nature of human life in the present moment. With no great expectation or sense of grief, when working closely with dementia-diagnosed residents they possess abundant patience and understanding.

Home health worker Sairose Kassan writes:

> Mrs. Sharpe is in the early stages of Alzheimer's and calls every day asking if it is Wednesday. Muriel goes to her home every Wednesday to play cards and to take her for a walk. Muriel's reward is the satisfaction she feels helping and the gratitude she receives from Mrs. Sharpe's family. Muriel has mentioned several times 'it's the smile on Mrs. Sharpe's face when I get there which makes my day!'

TODAY: *Appreciate life stages.*

What are the human service worker's tools? Linda LaPointe, a Colorado long-term care professional and author, writes about the caregiver's toolbox:

> Carpenters use tools. Chefs use tools. Dentists use tools. (Thinking of those just makes me drool!)
>
> So what tools do human service workers use?
>
> Human service staff are the only workers I know whose major tool is themselves.
>
> Your tool is YOU! The whole, entire, physical human being of you! Your heart, your brain, your voice. Your eyes, your ears, your body. You use your heart in your work daily. In fact, such a big heart is what drove you to human services in the first place! That provides you with compassion but not pity, sensitivity without overreaction, acceptance without judgment, empathy even when lacking understanding.

As you face this challenging day, take note of what tools you take out of your bag. Perhaps you will notice a shortage of tools, and decide it is time to learn some new skills and techniques? Perhaps you haven't fully called upon your pure heart, and that's why some assignments are tougher than others? Every moment provides a new opportunity to sharpen your tools and experience an even greater reward. Keep a light touch and trust yourself.

TODAY: *Use your tools.*

Families say thanks:

> I know how busy you are, yet you always take your time and make sure my mother never loses her dignity. You always remember that my mother is a human being. She is vulnerable and feels her dependency on others. You fulfill not only her basic needs, but also her need to feel cared for and safe.

> When you are getting my mother ready to lie down, you are considerate, gentle and careful. You make sure she's comfortable before she goes to sleep. I've seen you sit with a dying resident after your shift is over.

> I've seen you make phone calls for residents during your break time.

> You've called me on the phone just to tell me what a good mood my Mom was in that day.

> It's hard to put into words my appreciation for CNAs. Because I cannot be with my mother on a daily basis, I depend on their help. I am grateful to so many people involved in their care and value them all. They are always available with a smile and such a great attitude. They are terrific. Thank you for all your quality care!

Thanks to the extra efforts of Sister Del Ray, this praise from family members was collected and shared with the staff of St. Patrick's Residence in Naperville, Illinois.

Most days, nobody has time to gather compliments and hand them out. Most days, if you want to get a sense for how the job is going, you look into your resident's eyes. Or close your eyes and consult your heart.

TODAY: *Know you are appreciated.*

I am forever struck by the near limitless capacity of caregivers to care. A few years ago, I traveled with a group of 36 certified nursing assistants to the California state house in Sacramento. The CNAs wanted to talk with lawmakers about proposed legislation to increase fines levied against nursing facilities. At the end of a successful day, we sat around the hotel lobby and shared stories of home. Now it was time to talk about us: How many kids do you have? Do you live alone? Ever do any other kind of work?

To my amazement, I discovered a common theme in these caregivers' lives, which I had not seen before. Most of them had a disabled family member at home!

Tales of crippled husbands and handicapped children were told, and I didn't detect anyone was surprised but me. No one seemed overwhelmed or burdened, either. These women knew themselves and the strong call of the work. Personal experience had taught them the demands of the disabled, and they had gone into caregiving with open eyes. I quietly contemplated their lives: caring for eight or ten or more nursing home residents for eight or ten or more hours a day, only to go home to their own personal patients.

My contact with caregivers is a never-ending series of humbling events. Spending time with these California caregivers, the primary breadwinners for their families, was one such moment. Women of pure heart and soul, they had learned their trade at the bedside of a loved one. Regarding the experience as a great blessing, they had built careers of utter devotion.

TODAY: *Honor 24-hour caregivers.*

I spent an hour assisting Jim, a 75-year-old hospice patient suffering with bone cancer, through his evening rituals in preparing for bed. A retired minister, Jim had a beautiful faith he had shared with me on a number of evenings, in regard to his impending death. He always had a great number of questions about what he might expect physically and we were able to discuss such issues openly.

On this evening, as we did on many evenings, we prayed together, finishing with a blessing for peace of mind and heart. I assured Jim that all the hospice caregivers were there to assist him with whatever he might need and to feel free in asking for the same. As I prepared to leave, I asked, 'Is there anything else, Jim?'

He responded, 'You have spent enough time with me, go now to share your ministry with others.'

My eyes welled with tears. I have always felt nursing to be a ministry, rather than a 'job.' This was the very first time, however, in 35 years of nursing, that a patient has recognized verbally and openly what I have always seen as a calling.

Patients have given me many words of thanks and praise, but Jim's words continue to be the most special of my nursing career.

—Terry Bucher, founder and president of
Florida Association of Nurse Assistants

TODAY: *Share your ministry.*

Stories are told of heroic acts and superhuman strength, when an individual comes to the aid of a stranger and risks his or her life in the process. Pulling drivers from burning cars, rescuing children who've fallen through the ice, these members of the human family show us the capacity of a pure heart.

The day-to-day routine in a nursing facility or other health-care residence usually lacks such grand-scale disasters. Residents do choke or require CPR, but most shifts are a repetition of the same basic services delivered the past 365 days. Does this mean the tasks are any less heroic than those performed at highway accidents or natural disasters?

Serving others, be it in an emergency or at the bedside, an aide requires remarkable courage. To willingly be with another human being who is in pain, frightened, angry, or even dying takes a certain blend of characteristics. Such rescuers of the wounded must be gentle yet strong, able to think clearly while considering all the feelings swirling around the victim.

Writer and diarist Anais Nin wrote, "Life shrinks or expands in proportion to one's courage." I don't believe she was referring to the notoriety or public acclaim that comes from saving another person's life or any similar dramatic acts. Courage here refers to one's commitment to live a full life, to speak up, reach out, and grow beyond what's easy and familiar into the unknown.

As caregivers, courage kicks in when we volunteer to be trained in a new skill or to take care of a patient with a disability or diagnosis we've have never encountered. A certain bravery is required at these moments, when we choose to expand our relationship with the world.

The pure heart is always listening for the next call to duty. To not respond would be to become smaller and shrink in stature and self-confidence. For caregivers of compassion, there is no turning back, only expansion ahead.

TODAY: *Be courageous.*

Imagine being affiliated with 1600 CNAs in 39 states, who boast a combined contribution to long-term care of 35,000 years!

The Twenty Year Club is an honorary member organization for experienced nursing assistants who provide direct care in nursing homes, homes, hospices, or other long-term care services. Individual memberships are free.

In the year 2000, the following individuals held Club records: From Ohio, Margaret Fletcher, 48 years; Barbara Korecki, 47 years; Betty Brewer, 47 years; and Ivory Allen, 46 years. From Georgia, Margaret Peek, 55 years and Roberto Taloria, 47 years. From Virginia, Elsie Tisdale-Davis, 48 years.

Fifty-five years of dedication to others? How can any of us fully appreciate Margaret's incredible life, her pure heart? Founded by the National Network of Career Nursing Assistants, the TYC seeks to:

• recognize and validate nursing assistants who provide consistency and predictability to the people in their care

• identify and address training needs and other issues relative to experienced nursing assistants

• foster community understanding of the role, responsibility and value of experienced nursing assistants in long-term care

Who is eligible? Aides who have completed 20 or more years of service in long-term care, not necessarily in one place or at one time. Every fall a national award is presented in Washington, DC to a new member with the most years of experience.

Nominate pure hearts today for membership in the Twenty Year Club.

Twenty Year Club, Career Nurse Assistants' Program, Inc., 3577 Easton Road, Norton, Ohio 44203-5661.

TODAY: *Honor long-serving CNAs.*

Watching CNAs bathe and dress a resident, my whole notion of what it means to be related begins to blur. Families are the closest blood we have. Yet I have seen an equal if not greater level of familiarity and love between caregivers and their residents.

What is family? What does it mean to be related?

When Margie's daughter told her mom, "I'm engaged!" Margie felt joy and panic simultaneously. "She is going to marry into a wealthy family from New York City. What will we do about her wedding? We can't afford anything!"

With her husband no longer able to work, Margie still managed. The children were grown and on their own. Still, a nursing assistant's wages didn't allow for savings, let alone financing a wedding. Listening to Margie's worries, her coworkers stated the obvious: "We're your family, we'll help put this wedding together!"

Soon, lists were circulating around the building. Alice's mother made wedding cakes, and Barbie's son was a DJ. The social work and admissions staff said they would handle all the finger foods, and have a big cooking party at someone's home the day before the wedding. The wedding dress, bridesmaids' gowns and all the other details were handled the same way—by Margie's extended family. "Hey, we have to impress those out-of-state in-laws!" they grinned.

Chances are you've seen this same loving spirit where you work. Baby showers and fundraisers for sick children are commonplace. Working with caring people with pure hearts, the definition of family gets pretty broad.

Bless you!

TODAY: *Be family.*

In 1999, billions of dollars were spent internationally *out of fear* of the year 2000. Businesses prepared for the worst, worrying if they would be "Y2K Ready." Imagine the same world family effort, this time working *out of love* to unite forces and resources. What would it take to prepare our hearts for the best, to be "Today Ready?"

We can create this beautiful, peace-filled world community we imagine by adopting a simple practice designed by Tibet's exiled leader, His Holiness the Dalai Lama.

1. Spend five minutes at the beginning of each day remembering we all want the same things (to be happy and be loved) and we are all connected to one another.

2. Spend five minutes—breathing in—cherishing yourself; and, breathing out—cherishing others. If you think about people you have difficulty cherishing, extend your cherishing to them anyway.

3. During the day extend that attitude to everyone you meet. Practice cherishing the "simplest" person, as well as the "important" people in your life; cherish the people you love and the people you dislike.

4. Continue this practice no matter what happens or what anyone does to you. These thoughts are very simple, inspiring and helpful. The practice of cherishing can be taken very deeply if done wordlessly, allowing yourself to feel the love and appreciation that already exists in your heart.

When the world didn't come to an end on New Year's Eve 1999, shouts of relief were heard around the globe. We had united around preparing for the worst. Today, let us pledge to unite around preparing for the best with one message and one heart: cherish all life.

TODAY: *Prepare for the best.*

Hunting down hypocrisy seems to have become the new American pastime. The media loves nothing more than finding a supposed saint and exposing him as Satan.

I suppose crooked politicians first turned us on to this sport. Professing noble ideals of public service, they convinced us they cared about what is good and true, and then lived to prove otherwise. Human beings, by our nature, always carry this dark side with us. What makes some more criminal than others is an ability to control those impulses.

The practice of trapping celebrities and other well-known figures in hypocritical or compromising acts doesn't interest me. I have always preferred to trust others and be trusted. Living in this environment where catching phonies is common practice, our minds are conditioned to doubt others' intentions, to question their sincerity.

Many millennia ago, Confucius said, "If the will be set on virtue, there will be no practice of wickedness. Superior men, and yet not always virtuous, they have been, alas! But there never has been an inferior man who was at the same time virtuous." It seems hypocrisy has fascinated humanity for a long time!

Yes, man can be superior without being of a pure heart. But one cannot have a pure heart without being superior. Americans who wonder if good public servants do still exist, if there are beings alive who live by the golden rule, need only go to the nearest nursing home and meet the selfless staff.

Pay attention to your own actions and reactions. Live a life that is an open book, where those searching for hypocrisy will find nothing.

Today: *Live with a pure heart.*

We point to our heart when we are talking about how we feel. Speaking strictly from an anatomical perspective, our brain is actually the seat of emotions. Within the brain, the limbic system resides at the front of the head and governs our feelings. The hypothalamus is considered the site of pleasure, and its neighbor, the amygdala, the site of rage. Another part, the hippocampus, retrieves long-term memory from storage and turns short-term memories into long-term form.

For all we know about the brain, it still remains a mystery. While much knowledge about the brain has been gathered by physicians during surgeries and autopsies, observation of behavior is also a tremendously rich source of information about the workings of the brain.

Most of the people living in America's nursing homes have lost some of their mental capacity. Caring for residents with Alzheimer's guarantees an unpredictable workday. When we consider the number of emotional sites alone that could be damaged, it is no wonder each resident presents a brand new picture.

"I took care of this little lady who thought the nurses' station was a store, the dining room was a restaurant and that I was a maid," Audrey recalled. A CNA for 30 years, she has plenty of stories to tell. "She was always so concerned that I would get a tip, she would say, 'make sure you put all this on my tab.'" Audrey assured her she would.

Respecting the wishes of residents, regardless of how funny or strange they may seem, is the honorable thing to do. Whether the brain is firing properly or not is of no consequence to the resident who wants to make sure Audrey is treated well. At the very least, we must follow Audrey's example, and make sure residents are treated equally well. Feelings remain, and the pure heart continues to call out to others.

TODAY: *Respect wishes.*

Dawn Ward, a writer who has worked in a nursing home kitchen in northern Indiana for 32 years, recalls a favorite resident with great respect. Notice how she tells the story, her pure heart radiating above all else. Neither judge nor jury, Dawn lovingly captures another human being's one-of-a-kind qualities. We end up joining Dawn, missing Ksen Doi in the spring:

I remember Ksen Doi well. She was a Japanese resident; a little lady who understood English but didn't speak it. From her habits of saving things, we knew she had been through the depression and the war. She must have had a hard life growing up, as she really did save things, down to her toilet paper. If it wasn't soiled, she would spread it out on her bedspread to dry, and reuse it. We really are spoiled in this country, aren't we?!

Ksen rarely ventured out of her room. When she went to take a shower, she would peek into the hallway. If she thought no one looking, she would make a beeline across the hall, then come back the same way.

We have fire drills monthly, and once a coworker made a mistake with Ksen. Rather than gently approaching her and talking all the while, she grabbed her by the arm, not rough but gentle. Ksen responded with a karate chop to her stomach.

On the occasion she walked in the hallway, and you saw her and she saw you, she would greet you by folding her hands and bowing down.

In the springtime, she could be found going down the hallway, looking outside, seeing the flowers and trees bloom. It was obvious that spring was a favorite time of year.

Every spring I still see Ksen Doi in my mind, wandering through, looking at spring blooming outside.

TODAY: *See the unique.*

The week her mother died, Dolly was at the bedside around the clock. An executive who lived many states away, Dolly visited her mother for two years whenever she could, but this time, she wasn't visiting. She knew her mom was dying, and she was staying.

"Over the years, the family had done what we could to make her room seem like home. Her bulletin board was filled with pictures and cards," Dolly said.

During one shift, a caregiver came into the room to check on Dolly's mom. "It is great you can be here," the aide told Dolly, as they began to talk about her Mom's condition. "I've seen your picture on the wall."

"Who's in that photo?" the aide asked.

"I couldn't believe it! She was pointing to a picture of my mother. I put them up there so staff would talk to her about her life, and this woman didn't even know it was my mother!"

Focused on our tasks, it is quite easy to miss the obvious. Yes, it is important to make sure charting is up to date, medications properly dispensed, and patients turned. But it is also vital when caring for a patient to get to know who they are.

At Teresian House in Albany, NY, the facility has gone to great lengths to acquaint staff with the lives of their residents. Outside each patient's room, a large, glassed-in shadow box hangs, full of treasures and keepsakes from the resident's life. Touring the facility, I burst into tears at the poignant lives displayed in miniature. Pictures of beaming brides, New Year's toasts in top hat and tails and bronze baby booties vividly conveyed stories of full lives. Every nursing home should imitate this magnificent way of recognizing the individuals in their care.

TODAY: *Know your residents.*

When the English clergyman Augustus Hare (1792-1834) wrote these words, I don't think he had met many loving nurses and nurses' aides:

> We need not be afraid that we shall go too far in serving others. There is no danger that any of us will ever go too far in the work of active love. There is no likelihood that any of us will become too bountiful, too kind, too helpful to his neighbor.

Technically, I don't think I can quarrel with Rev. Hare's basic philosophy. The world is always in need of love, sweet love. But in some of the nursing homes I have visited, I have watched some of the tenderest of ministrations, usually reserved for mother and baby.

At 4 in the morning, I was setting up for an in-service for the night shift. I had a key to the building so I wouldn't disturb the few staff members and sleeping residents by banging on the door. Walking quietly down the hall to the classroom, I overheard an aide talking softly to one of her residents. "It is alright dear, I'm here. Don't worry sweetheart, everything is fine. I'll help you get to the bathroom and we'll get you all fixed up again. OK, honey?"

Across the country, regulators, owners and lawmakers sit in offices, trying to write regulations and job descriptions that will guarantee the kind of tender loving care I witnessed that night. (Well, some of the regulators might be working on the rule that prohibits staff from using terms of endearment with residents. I pity these individuals, having to create and enforce a policy that is a crime against humanity. We all want to be wakened with kindness and affection. I doubt many people can be found who prefer to hear sanitized words, stripped of warmth at 4 AM)

No amount of training or law can replace the pure heart for directing caregiver performance. Pay attention to the inherent goodness within. Strive to be too bountiful, too kind, too helpful.

TODAY: *Practice inherent goodness.*

"Our residents don't live in a facility; we work in their *home*." The plain, hand-lettered sign above the time clock was a powerful reminder to staff about the home's guiding philosophy.

My friend, artist Michael Gruteke, lived many years as a young adult in nursing homes. (Remember meeting Mike on May 29?) Mike has encouraged me to consider writing a book from the residents' point of view, going to facilities and interviewing people about living in an institution. "Find out what they think!" he says.

I've read a few limited studies on the preferences of nursing home residents. To the question, "What makes a good day for you?" the most frequent answer reported is simply, "Knowing who helps me get up in the morning."

Relationships are central to our well-being and sense of self. Even the shyest people relax and open up with a few dear friends. Human beings need to feel anchored in the lives of others. Listen to new people get to know each other. The first few minutes are spent searching for some common links. Sometimes finding they are fans of a common team is enough to create a bond.

I once got a ride from the airport to my car (parked at the train station in the next town) from a woman who mistakenly thought we were both friends with someone named Terry Lang. I can't reconstruct the conversation we had on the plane that led to the misunderstanding. As we talked, I remember being disarmed by her friendliness and generous offer to give me a ride. Later, as I got out of her car at the train station, she smiled and said, "Tell Terry I said 'hello!'" Hmmm.

Comforting connections, real, not imagined, are at the heart of a good day. While other factors, such as good food and personal privacy, also influence resident satisfaction, it is the close contact with one's caregiver that makes your facility a home. Be yourself. Others are waiting to know you!

TODAY: *Make the facility a home.*

Mildred was considered mean by nearly everyone who worked at Maple Lane. We weren't consciously looking for reasons to dislike her; she just kept committing nasty acts against other residents and staff.

The newest aide on the floor, I found that my inexperience infuriated Mildred, and she made her disgust well-known. "Have you ever dressed anyone before?" she would snap at me. Dependent on oxygen, she couldn't understand why I wouldn't turn the dials on the concentrator. "Give me more! I can't breathe!" she would scream, capping off her tirade with a few choice profanities.

I talked with other CNAs about Mildred; no one had any real insight into her life. A widow with no children, she had worked most of her life for the FBI and lived in Washington, D.C.

As I confessed that the only people I had ever dressed were my son and myself I noticed a moment of sadness move across Mildred's face. "We couldn't have a child," she told me, and she never learned why. She abruptly told me to leave the room, and returned to her grouchy self.

The next day, I brought a large picture of my son Elliot, taken when he was in first grade. "Elliot is now a teenager, Mildred, and it isn't easy. We could use your prayers. Can I leave this picture here to remind you?" Mildred brightened. She loved the idea.

My schedule changed at my other job, and I had to leave Maple Lane. I learned later of Mildred's death, and that Elliot's picture had remained with her. "I don't know where they sent her personal property," a former coworker told me, "but the picture went with it." As it should have.

TODAY: *Defuse the grouchy.*

Every profession has certain popular stories that circulate through the ranks. Call it mythology or hyperbole; these well-worn saws are passed on from veterans to the new hires, keeping old beliefs alive.

Direct care workers, who see themselves on the frontline doing the heavy lifting, wish management would walk a day in their shoes. "They don't have any idea how hard we work. Let them see what we do by doing it. I dare them to work one day on my job. They would see how hard it is."

Oh, if we could just get that administrator from behind the desk and onto the floor!

I doubt Bill Floyd had been on the job long enough to hear any of this nursing home oral history. The new chief executive officer and president of Beverly Healthcare, Mr. Floyd decided he wanted to work one week as a nursing assistant, to learn what his new company was all about. He said:

> One night, I worked alongside an aide while he helped a female resident get ready for bed. First he took off her artificial legs! Then he removed her wig. Once she was settled in bed, we started to leave the room to help someone else. I turned around for one last look. From her bed, this beautiful woman winked at me.

Hearing Bill Floyd's story, his caregiver audience nodded with deep appreciation and understanding. Despite the limitations and changes that come with old age, the human spirit remains. Within one wink we find an important lesson for all of us in the world of long-term care, including the decision-makers sitting at the desks.

TODAY: *Look for spirit.*

July: Blessed are the peacemakers, for they shall be called children of God

Peace is our natural state. Not stagnant, dormant or inert, peace is an active way of being. When we are living as designed, to be conscious is to be at peace. Peace is not only the absence of strife; it is also personal and global justice and joy.

Conflicts spring from being at odds with what we believe we are owed. Individuals who are not at peace see themselves as separate from others, different and somehow short-changed or hurt.

Peacemakers are healers, able to reach out and help others cooperate, to find their valued place in the human family. Always looking for commonalities, rather than differences, peacemakers draw people together for the greater good, recognizing all men as brothers and women as sisters.

Some say practicing peace is God's work, delegated to angels or divine beings. But we can all be peacemakers and enjoy the rewards. What is required is a peace-filled heart and a willingness to be motivated by trust, love and obedience.

Caregivers are naturally peacemakers because their most driving desire is to assure and restore well-being. Conflicts are resolved before they escalate, as the caregiver remains focused on returning everyone to this natural state.

Hidden in the shadows of warmakers who receive high honors, peacemakers are often unsung heroes. Taking a lesson from caregivers, world leaders need to become aware of their deep inner peace, and allow it to shape their actions. When humanity takes sides, everyone loses.

In the Mideast the Israelis pray for "shalom." The Arabs pray for "salom." Surely, sharing five of six letters makes these peoples more friends than enemies.

In the West we say to one another, "Peace be with you," meaning, "I surrender to you." Both parties surrender. Both are victorious. Both are blessed peacemakers.

"The meeting of two personalities is like the contact of two chemical substances: if there is any reaction, both are transformed," the psychotherapist Carl Jung wrote.

Transformed into what?

Nursing home civil wars are painful sieges. Night shift is mad at the day shift. Therapy is mad at nursing. And everyone is ticked off at how long maintenance takes to make repairs.

Patsy was a nursing assistant with a fierce grudge: "That director of nursing hated me, I know it. She never gave me a break. But if you were her pet, you had it made. I hate this place." Listening for a while, I learned Patsy's enemy DON had left three years ago. Yet Patsy was still angry!

If you've ever hugged someone who wasn't glad to see you, you know the lackluster feeling. Being a resident cared for by a disgruntled caregiver feels no better. "Oh, I hide it most days," Patsy told me of her rage, "I just thought you were someone I could tell."

Ask Patsy's residents, coworkers and even the visitors: mad attitudes can't be hidden. Too big and bulky, they leak out whenever an opportunity arises. Ask Patsy why she always feels tired and achy, sometimes with a new illness every week: mad attitudes suck the life out of everyone they touch.

If you're nursing an old wound, let it go. Make peace with the past and move on. Isn't it time to fully enjoy a brand new day, without yesterday's news clogging your ears and heart?

TODAY: *Make peace with the past.*

Caregivers can sometimes spend almost as much time caring for the resident's family members as for the actual resident. Struggling to accept the fact their loved one lives in a nursing home, relatives may need help finding peace. Family members of people living at St. Patrick's Residence in Naperville, Illinois are especially grateful for loving caregivers:

> You make me feel at peace. When I'm not here, I know my husband is in good hands.

> When I call and say, 'I can't make it today,' you say 'Don't worry, you know we take care of everything when you're not here.

> You have such a wonderful sense of humor. You are calm, gentle. I've never heard you raise your voice or act frustrated.

> I feel so good that my sister is with you. When she was home with me, I was worried. Now, I don't worry about her. She never complains here.

When one accepts the caregiver call and makes this work a career, the labels people carry matter little. Wherever there is need for reassurance and ease, the loving caregiver steps forward. The distinctions of "resident" and "family member" are secondary. What's primary in the heart and soul of the peacemaking caregiver is knowing a human being needs soothing.

TODAY: *Help families find peace.*

For the Tsaligi (Cherokee) as with many other American Indian nations, care of elders is important to our understanding and survival as a people. Elders teach us the right way to do things, and to not take ourselves too seriously. Life is meant to be fun in the learning experiences we are given by the Creator; I admit many times I take things in the wrong way.

As humans, we are not perfect, that is why we are constantly learning. It is also important we look not at the color of one's skin, but at a person's heart and soul. Treating others as we would like to be treated is very important to how I do my job as a nursing assistant, for one day it may be me who is that elderly resident and I hope I am cared for in a respectable loving manner. My parents have said, "The Wind comes around," so I hope my wind is a caring, warm one.

Each of us is a healer in a way, whether of others or ourselves. The elderly have given so much. It is important I give and help them as they complete their life path. Even the way we approach dying is a lesson in life for us to understand. My ancestors cried at births and rejoiced at deaths. Today if you attend a traditional Tsaligi funeral, it starts at sunrise and goes until sunset, with food, drumming, singing, and telling of "remember when" stories.

Many times a giveaway of the person's belongings also occurs at that time, although this can occur up to one year later. The giveaway is a way to help others as well as for the family to heal.

Learning and understanding is a way of healing others and ourselves. Healing is not just putting a band-aid on a visual sore; people have invisible sores from past hurts. I hope my interaction with others is done in such a way that I help them heal invisible hurts. Hurts come from many sources; many are part of our childhood and go into adulthood, and we repeat the same lessons over and over again until we can pass that test, then graduate onto the next class of life.

We need to forgive the past and learn from the mistakes we make in our lives to help us grow into the special people we can become. We are not perfect, but we can strive to be the very best we can be, doing the right thing at the right time, in the right way. This is the path of beauty, an interior beauty that my heritage teaches so strongly.

—Valerie Cooper, CNA, Birmingham, Alabama. A Native American, she writes under the name Bull Star.

TODAY: *Do the right thing at the right time in the right way.*

Living or working alone, we can ignorantly imagine we are calm and peaceful individuals, just harmless pussycats. Introduce another person into our space, though, and watch the catfight commence! And being perfect, we decide it isn't our fault the fur flew.

As any preschooler knows, getting along with others and learning to share isn't easy. Alone, we are what we are. But in community, we are in relation to others.

Besides potential conflicts, groups also present us with the chance to become our whole selves. Passive individuals learn to become assertive, and the domineering learn to listen. If we don't learn we remain opposites, the passive become victims and the domineering the perpetrators.

According to the Bahá'í faith's teachings, universal peace will be triggered, in part, by the linking together of polar opposites:

> The East is in need of material progress and the West is in need of a spiritual ideal. It would be well for the West to turn to the East for illumination and to give in exchange its scientific knowledge. There must be this interchange of gifts. The East and the West must unite to give each other what is lacking. This union will bring about true civilization where the spiritual is expressed and carried out in the material. Receiving thus, the one from the other, the greater harmony will prevail, all people will be united, a state of great perfection will be attained, there will be a firm cementing, and this world will become a shining mirror for the reflection of the attributes of God. (Excerpted from The Bahá'ís, a publication of the Bahá'í International Community.)

We can use this recipe for peace in the workplace by consciously exchanging gifts with our opposites. If you are a poor bed-maker, find the champion in your ranks and ask for lessons. By sharing your strengths, a state of perfection will be attained and peace will prevail.

TODAY: *Share your gifts.*

My mother and I have a joke about "the boy at camp." Though we went to camp in different times and places, we both thought the one boy who worked at our all-girls' camp was just gorgeous. Seeing these guys in the fall, in the company of classmates, we wondered, "What were we thinking?"

The isolated environment of any institutional setting can throw off our judgment. Consider the number of office romances; proximity surely makes the heart grow fonder. Love isn't the only threat to a level head when we spend a lot of time in one place. Hate is equally attractive and easy to whip up. The controlling force is the Closeness Factor. Finding the right balance, when someone isn't too close or too far away, is a critical assignment for peacemakers.

Drivers who see life as a contest hate other drivers with little effort. I call it long-distance hating: at a certain distance, drivers freely yell and scream at one another, making rude hand gestures and facial expressions. But as the distance shortens, most are less brave and dramatic. The Closeness Factor determines behavior.

Life is not a sport. If any metaphor could apply, it would be the dance. For everyone to have a good time, we need to give one another space and avoid stepping on toes. Become aware of the unique challenges presented by confining and crowded spaces, and be better prepared to keep the peace.

TODAY: *Dance in your space.*

Nancy lived a sheltered life before she became a nursing assistant. Caring for grandparents and parents at home, she married late and had her children even later. She became a widow early.

"Taking care of people was all I knew," she said, explaining why she became an aide. A reserved, shy woman, Nancy had seen little of the world. Receiving her first paycheck the month she turned 50 was a momentous occasion.

Though she loved her residents dearly, Nancy found some of the nursing staff to be bullying and difficult. She felt she got a raw deal on scheduling. They said, "You've got no one at home, so you can work Christmas." A devout Roman Catholic, Nancy wanted to go to church at Christmas, but she always had to work the holiday.

Her daughters, all working women, told her to "fight for her rights." Nancy confided in her closest friend at work, worried she wouldn't be able to muster up the self-confidence for a fight.

"Nancy, this is not about fighting," Janice told her. "This is about standing up for yourself, and being responsible. We don't need another nasty fighter here, believe me!"

As caregivers, our actions should spring from peace-filled hearts. Giving voice to violence, for whatever purpose, poisons the planet. Nancy had to make a logical case for her position, not an angry, emotional appeal. Showing others how to advocate for change without criticizing is the job of each peacemaker. We don't need to be a bad guy in order make our point.

TODAY: *Stand up and be responsible.*

I'm surprised healthcare facilities don't have staff filing worker's compensation claims for being strangled by the rumor grapevine. Keeping up with the latest version of the truth can be a full-time job.

Rita found herself the subject of some hot gossip, and got ticked off. "I told the director of nursing that someone had tied up the nurses' station telephone for 15 minutes with a personal call. I knew she was wrong, but it wasn't my job to discipline, so I reported it."

In handling the problem, the administrator made a big goof: she told Judy, the offending nurse, that Rita had reported her. "I thought I was mad, but Judy was out of control," Rita said, describing the campaign of retaliation that ensued. Judy turned her head whenever Rita walked down the hall.

A mutual friend told Rita what was going on. "You've got to make peace with her, Rita," their friend said. "We can't live with this tension, everyone feels it." Rita confided that she was starting to dread coming to work, and had been having trouble sleeping. "I can't live with this either!"

At her friend's insistence, Rita went to Judy with a "peace offering." "Judy accepted the offering relatively well, though she is still convinced I said something derogatory about her. I told her I did not, but that was actually beside the point. I said I did not want this misunderstanding to interfere with the working relationship that we must maintain and she agreed," Rita told her friend.

What is commendable about Rita's actions is her willingness to make the first move. How many of us say, "I'll apologize, but first she needs to apologize to me!" "Only when you have made peace within yourself will you be able to make peace in the world," is wise advice from Rabbi Simcha Bunim.

By being a peacemaker, Rita advanced the healing.

TODAY: *Make the first move for peace.*

In Sunday school, I remember singing this every week:

Friends, friends, friends. I have some friends I love. I share my games and share my toys, with all my friends both girls and boys. Friends, friends, friends. I have some friends I love.

Songs and stories are great ways to communicate. I especially like this little tale from Vietnam, and encourage you to share it in the practice of peacemaking:

The Vietnamese believe that after death people go to heaven or hell. Hell, according to legend, is where you are given a 50-foot banquet table with all of your most favorite foods in abundant quantities. Residents of hell are given three-foot chopsticks, so they can reach the food but not their mouths.

Heaven-bound, in the Vietnamese belief system, the deceased finds the same bounteous table and the same three-foot chopsticks. The only difference is that in heaven, the residents feed each other.

So where do you work? Heaven or Hell?

TODAY: *Make a heavenly home.*

Caregivers are asked to do many things for residents; the list is never-ending. Sometimes, frightened family members ask for miracles. "What can you do to make my mother well? She is so weak," they cry, and your heart breaks for them.

Leaving the rooms of these patients and families, the peace-making caregiver says, "I'll be back. Everything is OK, I'll come and check on you again." Of course, these are the words of peace.

For your Jewish residents, consider offering a healing prayer in their tradition. Why not invite the family to recite the Mi Shebeirach Prayer for Healing with you? Ask for help with pronunciation; they will be thrilled to teach you.

> O God, who blessed our ancestors, Abraham, Isaac and Jacob, Sarah, Rebekah, Rachel and Leah, send your blessings to (NAME OF RESIDENT). Have mercy on him/her, and graciously restore his/her health and strength. Grant him/her a R'fua Shleima (a complete recovery), a R'fuat Hanefesh (a healing of spirit), and a R'fuat Haguf (a healing of body)—along with all others who are stricken. May healing come speedily, and let us say: Amen.

TODAY: *Pray for healing.*

Nearing his 100th winter, Passaconaway, the Great Chief and Medicine Man of the Penacooks (one of the Abenaki Groups) issued a warning at a great gathering of New England tribes. It was 1665, on the plains above Concord, New Hampshire.

The Warning of 1655

I am an old oak that has lasted the storms of many winters. My eyes are dim and my limbs tremble. The scalplocks that dried before my wigwam told the stories of my victories over the Mohawks who invaded our hunting grounds. Then, in their place, came the Palefaces. The lands of our forefathers were taken from us...I tried the magic of my sorcery in vain...Now, my children, heed my dying words. The oak will soon break before the whirlwind...I commune with the Great Spirit. He whispers to me, 'Tell your people, peace. Peace is your only hope...your forests shall fall before their mighty hatchets. At your fishing places, they shall build their houses!' We must bend before the storm...Peace, peace with the White man is the command of the Great Spirit, and the last wish of Passaconaway.

As I type these words, I sit in my northern Vermont home, on land that was once home to the Abenaki people. Quite possibly, the first farming done on our 160 acres was done by white settlers who stole the land from the Abenakis.

No, I did not inherit the land; I have no relationship with any prior owners. Still, I wonder about my responsibility today, owning stolen property. Art seized by the Nazis is being returned to the ancestors of the burglarized owners. Pope John Paul has apologized to the Jews for past acts of the Catholic Church. A late reconciliation or apology is better than none.

Become aware of the injustices and wrongs suffered by those in your care. Listen to the stories they repeat, of unfair treatment and worse at the hands of another human being.

As a peacemaker, on behalf of the human race, past present and future, apologize. Let them know you believe their experience was awful and undeserved. Work for peace.

TODAY: *Apologize for inhumanities.*

A neighbor once told us his dad had a private plane. His announcement unleashed a pack of questions, the most frequent being, "Can we see it? Can we go for a ride?"

The poor kid had made up the plane, and made up plenty of answers before the whole story crashed and burned. As Shakespeare tells us, "What a tangled web we weave when first we practice to deceive."

Have you noticed that afternoon soap operas are almost exclusively based on one theme: deception? Characters hold a secret and worry their secret will be revealed. If each one just told the truth, the shows would be canceled.

Lives based on deception and dishonesty cause great grief. Talk about disturbing the peace! Something smells rotten, but no one can figure it out. Like the little boy with his father's pretend plane, we can say things that aren't true without wanting to do any harm.

I suspected a woman friend was beaten by her husband. When we had to share a room during a convention, I confirmed my suspicions. While she first tried to convince me she had simply fallen, Marlene eventually told the whole horrid story in her frightened little voice. Now, her tardiness and unpredictability made sense. Marlene wasn't a bad employee, she was a battered wife! I firmly told her she deserved peace and that I would not rest until she agreed. With the deception over, together we found her a safe home and Marlene began a new life.

TODAY: *Tell the truth.*

Pause to reflect on the countless times your hands have gently cared. Dr. Jane Thibault of the University of Louisville writes:

> Your hands are the ambassadors of your inner self. They manifest your thoughts, your feelings, your creativity, your destructiveness, your love, your hate, your unity to others, and your isolation. When you hold the hand of a frail resident, you are affirming your willingness to share her pain...Let us be willing to become aware of how we love the world through our hands. Through them we are truly the creative fingertips of the Creator; we allow creation to continue, to unfold through us.

Isn't it time to pay tribute to your precious hands?

Blessed be the works of your hands, O Holy One.
Blessed be these hands that have touched life.
Blessed be these hands that have nurtured creativity.
Blessed be these hands that have held pain.
Blessed be these hands that have embraced with passion.
Blessed be these hands that have tended gardens.
Blessed be these hands that have closed in anger.
Blessed by these hands that have planted new seeds.
Blessed be these hands that have harvested ripe fields.
Blessed be these hands that have cleaned, washed, mopped and scrubbed.
Blessed be these hands that have become knotty with age.
Blessed be these hands that are wrinkled and scarred from doing justice.
Blessed be these hands that have reached out and been received.
Blessed be these hands that hold the promise of the future.
Blessed be the works of your hands, O Holy One.

—Diann Neu

TODAY: *Arrange for a hand blessing.*

Zen teacher Bernie Glassman has described the mystical tradition that is your ancestry:

> In most mystical traditions, the role of the mystic, the peacemaker, is to make whole. Making peace is making whole...The word peacemaker in Hebrew is two words: Oseh Shalom. Oseh: maker. Shalom: peace. The Jewish mystics like to move around the vowels of a root word and see what emerges. If you do that to the root of Shalom, you get Shalem, which means whole. To make peace means to make whole.

> Making peace, making things whole, is an endless task. There are many definitions of a peacemaker. One of these I like most is that a peacemaker, knowing that the well needs water, climbs the mountain to reach the snow, gets a spoonful of snow, comes down, drops it in the well, and goes back up the mountain. She knows the task is endless but she does as much of it as she can, day after day after day.

> Making peace, yes, its overwhelming. That's why we never stop doing it. The reason we get overwhelmed is that we want to achieve a certain goal. If we aren't attached we wouldn't be overwhelmed. It's endless. And we just take one step after the next.

Caregivers tend to be unaware of or diminish their role in the history of the world. As peacemakers, you are to heal and make whole.

TODAY: *Heal and make whole.*

(Reprinted from *Bearing Witness: A Zen Master's Lessons in Making Peace* by Bernie Glassman. New York, Harmony Books. Copyright © 1998 p. 71.)

Ever overhear gossip or receive a tongue-lashing? Or worse, have you given one? I write "worse" because being the perpetrator is a greater burden to bear.

I once overheard two people talking about me. I had traveled to Washington, DC for a three-day healthcare convention which required lots of preparation. Not only did I have to make arrangements for my son's care, but I had to get ahead at work to avoid a backlog when I returned. Arriving at the hotel, I was exhausted. The last thing I wanted to do was go party. I figured the first swallow of wine would knock me out. Roll call was at 8 AM, so I gave my regrets to the group and headed for bed.

Unaware I was still waiting for the elevator, two board members stood behind a hotel pillar and ran me down: "She gets all the way down here and she wants to eat in her room? What the hell is the matter with her? What do we pay her for?"

Back in my room, I slammed my pillow around, had a few tears and fell asleep. Years later, I discovered this Proverb, and decided to look up various translations. Pick your favorite and post it on the refrigerator at home, to remind you to use your tongue as an instrument of peace.

Proverbs 15:4

A soothing tongue is a tree of life, But perversion in it crushes the spirit.

—New American Standard

A gentle tongue is a tree of life, but perverseness in it breaks the spirit.

—New Revised Standard

Kind words bring life, but cruel words crush your spirit

—Good News Bible

A soothing word is a staff of life, but a mischievous tongue breaks the spirit.

—New English

The tongue that soothes is a tree of life; the perverse tongue, a breaker of hearts.

—The New Jerusalem Bible

Gentle words cause life and health; griping brings discouragement.

—Living Bible

A soothing word is a tree of life, but a mischievous tongue breaks the spirit.

—Revised English

A wholesome tongue is a tree of life, but perverseness in it breaks the spirit.

—New King James

TODAY: *Make your tongue an instrument of peace.*

The Lenni Lenape (Delaware) was a Native American tribe with peaceful inclinations. The Lenape were known as mediators and peacemakers in colonial America. Their reputation for mediation or peacemaking was associated with the name "Gantowises"—meaning "women"—which they accepted for themselves.

Some scholars believe this name was a badge of honor, originating with Iroquois women of royal lineage who had a highly honored role as peacemakers. The term "Gantowises" lost status when translated into the English, because the English had no equivalent role of honor for women.

Being called a peacemaker is a badge of honor. When the first volume of *For Goodness' Sake* was published, my editor, Dr. David Bryan, suggested I find a famous caregiver to write the introduction. "A well-known person will advance sales," he explained.

"A famous caregiver? Who would that be?" I asked.

After a long pause, he said somewhat sheepishly, "Dr. Quinn, medicine woman?" I dismissed this fictional character. He then went through a list of dead women, including Clara Barton and Florence Nightingale. "How about Dear Abby?" he asked rather lamely.

"David, you're pointing out exactly why I wrote this book. We don't elevate caregivers to celebrity status. We lift up the names of parents who kill their children and children who murder their classmates. Let us hope society becomes aware of the majesty of the peacemaking caregiver."

TODAY: *Be a Gantowise.*

Peacemaking isn't overlooking conflict. Overlooking conflict is just that: pretending, hoping it will magically disappear like dust bunnies under the bed.

When we are angry with someone, we think staying angry, but hiding it, is an option. It isn't. We can't hide it, because anger has one goal: to express itself.

Another option is to just let the anger go, without any more thought or wasted time—a noble approach, but rarely possible.

Yet another option is to work on determining the underlying reason you're angry and work through it. Sorting and sifting through anger requires gentleness with oneself.

When I sit quietly and review why my husband steamed my rice, I recall old, similar stories with other men, going right back to my father. Maybe it is time to get rid of the goat I keep inside so men can't get it anymore! I also hold out—that is, I let go of most of my fury, but I still cling to some little fact that makes me ambivalent and unable to move on. "Maybe he was a jerk!" I think, remaking the arguments in my head for why I have a right to be angry.

Overlooking conflict or holding on to conflict won't work. To make peace, we have to work it through and let it go. With such short lifetimes, we must concentrate on letting go. Forgive yourself and the Other. Then move on and have some fun.

TODAY: *Forgive and have fun.*

Try to do everything with a mind that lets go. Do not expect any praise or reward. If you let go a little, you will have a little peace. If you let go a lot, you will have a lot of peace. If you let go completely, you will know complete peace and freedom. Your struggles with the world will have come to an end.

Maybe that was easy for the late Buddhist monk, Ajahn Chah, to write, but it is not easy for me to live! At the risk of great oversimplification, Buddhism teaches us three truths about suffering: all men suffer; we suffer because of our attachments; and the way to end suffering is to end attachments.

A fellow Vermonter, Ann Cason, has written a wonderful book for families called *Circles of Care: How To Set up Quality Home Care For Our Elders* (Shambala Boston, 2001). A caregiver and Buddhist, she wrote of her own father's aging:

My father was an entrepreneur who pioneered new products and developed many businesses. Work had been his life. His pleasure was getting up early and writing out his plans and dreams on yellow pads. When he lost his health, he had to give up his business. His memory failed, and he lost his ability to be a provider. He had always been cheerful and optimistic when facing big obstacles in life, but this time he sank and couldn't recover.

He began to spend his days sitting in an easy chair watching television. Since he could no longer drive, his second wife Eleanor, fifteen years younger and still working, had to leave her job every time he needed to go to the doctor or wanted to go swimming. The only stimulation my father could find in his narrowing world was trying to win millions of dollars from *Reader's Digest* or Publisher's Clearing House.

As I looked at the way my father lived his life, I was filled with tenderness and fear and the heart-wrenching desire to fix it. At the same time, I respected the way he was managing. He had been such a doer, always making things happen, and now he was up against something very basic. He—and I—had to learn to be with his life as it was.

He and I had to learn to be with his life as it was. As caregivers, if we can let go completely, we can know complete peace and freedom.

TODAY: *Let go and know peace.*

(From *Circles of Care* by Ann Cason. Copyright © 2001 by Ann Cason. Reprinted by arrangement with Shambhala Publications, Inc., Boston, www.shambhala.com)

She is a nursing assistant I regard with the greatest affection and admiration, but I cannot use her name. She maintains stories of her gracious heart can "get her in trouble," so she asks me not to use her name. I will call her Grace.

When a charge nurse, in the presence of other staff, verbally dressed down a newly certified aide, Grace experienced the event as hurting everyone. Rather than taking sides or making judgments, she saw the damaged soul of the charge nurse, the frightened spirit of the new hire and the anxious uneasiness of the spectators. Grace said:

> I told the staff who heard it to one by one, quietly, take the new girl aside and support her. Tell her that what happened wasn't right, that no one deserved to be treated that way, that no one had the right to treat another person that way. I also asked them to compliment her work and let her know that she was really becoming a good aide.

The next day, Grace brought a flowering plant to the charge nurse who had blown up at the young aide. Placing the plant into the nurse's hands, Grace said, "Something must be going on in your life to have caused that scene yesterday in the hall. I know you are a good person." Accepting the plant, the nurse burst into tears, saying, "How could you be so kind to me? I am a *****."

In the words Mahatma Gandhi, the man who led his nation of India from British rule to freedom without violence, "Leadership at some time meant muscles; but today it means getting along with people."

Grace is a magnificent example of loving leadership, making peace without taking sides.

TODAY: *Get along.*

In France in 1964, with Rapha'l Simi and Philippe Seux, two men with developmental disabilities, Jean Vanier founded L'Arche, a community of men and women who have developmental disabilities. From this original community, 103 other communities have been founded throughout the world, in Europe, Africa, Asia, North and South America.

From their web site, www.larchecanada.org:

> L'Arche (the Ark) is about life sharing, revealing the unique value of people. L'Arche is about living out spirituality in a very concrete way. L'Arche is about long-term commitment to each other and changing society, by being a sign of hope and love.

What makes L'Arche homes different from other residences that serve people with disabilities is that everyone lives under one roof, caregivers included. Basing community life on living the Beatitudes, Vanier offers six ways to be a peacemaker:

1-respect every individual human being
2-create space for people to grow and mature
3-always stay in dialogue
4-keep adapting mutual expectations
5-enjoy the differences between people
6-always direct your attentions to those who suffer most

Reflecting on an interaction at a L'Arche home in Canada, an anonymous caregiver said:

> Always my problem with Paul was the same: why couldn't he shower after a day working on the farm? I couldn't enjoy my meal sitting next to someone who smelled like a barnyard. Paul's view was that if this was his home, he could be comfortable in his own way after a hard day's work.

> One night at the dinner table, Paul's smell and my annoyance grew so intense that after a loud argument Paul angrily left the table. The rest of us tried to recreate some feel of family sharing. After dishes, Frank

called me aside to his bedroom where I could understand him despite his speech difficulties. 'I see you're
having trouble with Paul,' he said carefully. I brushed
his concern aside, 'Never mind. Paul and I will work it
out.' Frank looked me in the eye and said, 'You know, if
you want to help Paul, you have to start loving him.'

TODAY: *Start by loving.*

Visiting from Scotland, Heather envied Vermont's short growing season, the very growing season my husband and I regularly curse! "Our gardens last so long, everything gets leggy and the weeds take over!" Heather said, extolling the advantages of our short-lived garden.

"But we spend all summer worrying the frost will come before the harvest!" I told her, joking it seems even the garden is greener on the other side of the ocean.

Looking at the events of another place or time, it is human nature to conclude that our own circumstances are lacking. But what if these conclusions aren't right, and neither circumstance is any better or worse? What if, regardless of the century or the location, the challenges of human existence are essentially the same? Could it be that, despite all of the technological and material advances, the experience of being human is virtually unchanged?

Caregivers have been part of every civilization, the glue holding communities together. I imagine children of the nomadic people who lived long before the time of Christ needed to hear the reassuring voice of their mothers when they woke at night. I expect the sick and dying longed for a cool drink of water and a gentle touch as well.

As an experiment, listen for comments that suggest conditions are worse here and now compared to something else. Help yourself and others to recognize the humor in such comparisons, pointing out that human beings are forever thinking their lot is worse. As peacemakers and healers, part of your call is to remind others of life's opportunities, and to provide reasons for hope and joy. "Be among those who renew this world and bring prosperity and solace to creation." Zarathushtra wrote that bit of inspiration about 1738 B.C. His visitors probably envied his garden, too!

TODAY: *Renew hope and bring solace.*

On payday, Ben buys lottery tickets. Wednesday nights, Alice plays bingo. Saturday mornings, Dave washes his car while his wife washes the dog.

Routines keep us grounded and organize our lives. Possibilities for designing meaningful moments in our day are limitless. With so much structure imposed by the demands of work and home, the idea of willingly adding yet another regular task or assignment can seem pretty unappealing. But wait! Setting aside precious time for yourself isn't cause for rebellion.

Within the Zen Peacemaker Order members around the world stop at noon for one minute of silent meditation for world peace. Practitioners find great strength in this unified effort. Instead of seeing themselves as isolated individuals who work to reduce violence, associates of this Buddhist group symbolically join hearts daily, in the name of peace.

What simple gestures could you include in your day to magnify peace and link yourself to kindred spirits? The frequent use of guns by children is reason enough to establish a caregiver ritual in your place of work or community at large. Could all caregivers say a silent prayer for valuing life whenever they hear a bell ring? What a loving force you could generate.

TODAY: *Create a peacemaking ritual.*

A Vision of Hope

> We pray that someday an arrow will be broken, not in something or someone, but by each of humankind, to indicate peace, not violence.
>
> Someday, oneness with creation, rather than domination over creation, will be the goal to be respected.
>
> Someday fearlessness to love and make a difference will be experienced by all people.
>
> Then the eagle will carry our prayer for peace and love, and the people of the red, white, yellow, brown and black communities can sit in the same circle together to communicate in love and experience the presence of the Great Mystery in their midst.
>
> Someday can be today for you and me. Amen.

—Wanda Lawrence, Chippewa, 20th century

The image of breaking an arrow before it is used as a weapon is mighty. When my son was little, he loved carrying his squirt gun on walks. From the beginning, I explained he could not point the gun at living things. One Saturday in front of the post office, aiming at the flag pole, he hesitated and said, "Mom, is that a loving thing?"

Long before you do injury to another person by whispering cruelties or being mean-spirited, remember s/he is a loving thing. Break your arrow before it is used as a weapon.

TODAY: *Break arrows before use.*

I first saw a sign about guns in a nursing home in 1999. "No guns in facility" was posted on the back door of a facility outside of Atlanta.

Prior to that summer, the concept had never entered my consciousness. A few months later, I read that the United Nations estimated more than 500 million guns and other small arms were circulating around the world, widely used because they are lethal, inexpensive, easy to care for and hide.

"We have been concerned that a lot of folks don't see gun violence as their problem; they see it as someone else's problem," said gun violence researcher Philip Cook, director of the Sanford Institute of Public Policy at Duke University.

A study estimated the annual cost of treating gunshot victims in the U.S. is more than $2.3 billion. Government pays half of that bill. As taxpayers fund government, the author concluded, "We all have a stake in reducing gun violence."

Gun violence is absolutely our problem, and for a far greater reason than simply sharing the victims' medical bills: we are members of this troubled human race! Guns devalue life, cheapening its preciousness. We pay dearly for this damage. Nightly news programs (Dan, Peter and Tom's Atrocity Roundups) relentlessly remind us that we live in ever more violent world. Where is the voice of the peacemaker?

Where are you? Your colleagues? Daily you bring balance and ease to those in your care. In the face of constant confusion and conflict, caregivers apply healing balm. You soothe the anxious and angry brow. You are masters at guiding others away from violence. Can you teach the rest of us about making peace?

TODAY: *Teach peacemaking.*

Man's history has been one of battles. Woman's history has been that of hearing and raising children. Battles do not require any of the virtues needed for child raising— such as selfless and devoted love, compassion, benevolence, affection, gentleness and patience. On the contrary, these virtues are in the way on the battlefield. If, during a battle, love and benevolence toward the enemy rise in the heart, there won't be a battle. War requires hatred, anger, fear, cruelty, conquest and destruction.

Powerful words from Masami Saionji, chairperson of The World Peace Prayer Society. The Society is a nonprofit, member-supported, non-sectarian organization dedicated to spreading the message and prayer May Peace Prevail on Earth.

Through the Peace Pole Project, World Peace Prayer Ceremonies, the Peace Pals program for young people, and other initiatives, Society members and supporters around the world are working together to carry the universal message of peace to their communities on every continent. Founded in Japan in 1955, the Society has its world headquarters in New York City, and is affiliated with the Department of Public Information at the United Nations. You can find them on the Internet at www.worldpeace.org.

Descended from the Royal Ryukyu Family of Okinawa, Masami Saionji and her husband Hiroo Saionji have traveled around the world leading World Peace Prayer Ceremonies in many countries. How did she become involved in her vocation? A near-death experience as a young person led her to dedicate her life to world peace and humanity. She urges women to take an active role in the peace process:

> Since the world's history has evolved as man's history of war, the human race is far from attaining peace. For this very reason, women have to truly awaken and then, for the first time, they can make the world peaceful. World peace depends on each woman's merciful heart.

TODAY: *Depend on your merciful heart.*

One measure of world progress is man's insatiable desire for more. Greed rules so many transactions and actions.

Today I watched the morning talk show Regis and Kelly, a light television program that features what's new in fashion, music and film. I call it my brain flush. If I had a nearby neighbor, this would be time to share coffee, but since I don't, I watch a bit of TV.

In the middle of chatter about the weather, Regis took us live to the floor of the New York Stock Exchange to see how the market was performing! Is there no escaping this tendency to hitch our moods and attitudes to the Dow Jones Index?

Last night, a friend mentioned the American habit of rating a job by how much money one earns. "I've always valued time over money," he said. "I rate jobs by how much time they leave me for myself."

Peacemakers assess jobs based on how much healing is possible and how much good they can do. Once you realize you are a peacemaker, the way you see yourself and your work changes. No longer are you the lowest-paid healthcare worker, or as one depressed CNA once told me, the "butt wiper."

By what names and labels do you know yourself? Do you accept the identity known by your heart, or do you let the wealth-obsessed world minimize your greatness?

The ancient Hindu teachings, the Svetasvatara Upanishads, tell the story of the two birds that are inseparable friends, perched on the same tree. One bird eats the fruit; the other looks on without eating. The two birds are actual symbols representing the same person, the individual and the true Self. The individual eats the fruit of this world and gets tangled in all of the illusions or the maya, (see January 12) thinking s/he is a separate being. But when this self recognizes the other is the true Self, it is set free.

When the self forgets its true nature and gets immersed in this world, it is full of misery. When it recognizes its true Self, in the Lord, dwelling in the heart, then it attains peace.

Above all, let nothing make you forget your true nature. You are not chasing fame, fortune or power. You are here to make peace.

TODAY: *Know your true nature.*

Anthropologist Helen Fisher wrote:

> Holding grudges is probably an ancient practice among humans—female chimpanzees also nurse their grievances. Male chimps tend to make peace with one another within hours after a fight. But when a female is betrayed by another female who has handled her infant carelessly or eaten too much of the communal lunch, she may slap or shove the transgressor, then ignore her for days or weeks.

> When girls and women feel snubbed, they often stop speaking to you—unlike boys and men, who tend to express themselves with direct physical confrontation. Women exclude a colleague from informal meetings, ignore him or her at conferences and other business gatherings, and use their connections to present a united front against him or her.

In short, men stab you in the front while women prefer the back.

Front or back, stabbing isn't the way to deal with conflict. Unfortunately, both confrontation and shunning are common visitors at humanity's table. As peacemakers we have a duty to not seat these mischiefs in our homes or workplaces.

Keeping the peace and ending skirmishes is an art. We can't be intolerant. Foremost and always, be the presence of justice and kindness. When you learn of grudges and feuds, help free those caught in these angry traps. As the only animal with speech, we should be able to work things out more effectively than the chimps and apes!

TODAY: *Free the trapped.*

(Reprinted from *The First Sex: The Natural Talents of Women and How They are Changing the World* by Helen Fisher. New York, Ballantine Books. Copyright © 1999 p. 44.)

In the 1400's, before Englishmen set eyes on North America, an Iroquois League of Peace was formed. The League was an experiment in replacing violence with nonviolence. Its founding prophet was Deganawidah, a Huron by birth and a Mohawk by adoption.

Deganawidah came preaching a gospel of peace to the Iroquois during a time of great inter-tribal violence and war. The people should stop killing each other, he asserted, accept the rule of law, and come together in new rituals of unity.

Legend tells how Deganawidah recruited and converted three key persons who were caught up in the old way of violence, and invested them with positions of authority in the new, peaceful order. The new chiefs' council tackled the issue of disarmament and, at Deganawidah's suggestion, uprooted a great pine tree and threw all of their arms into the hole. Then they replanted the tree, "thus hiding the weapons of war forever from the sight of future generations."

The pine tree was a great symbol of unity. The Deganawidah epic is distinctive from the chartering myths of other nations because it found its unity in remembering the establishment of internal peace, rather than in celebrating triumphal military victory over threatening external enemies.

What are the weapons of war at your workplace? Gossip, sarcasm, profanity, unkindness, laziness? What about ganging up on others? Cliques?

Over coffee with coworkers, share this story and bravely suggest it is time to bury the weapons.

TODAY: *Bury the weapons.*

Redheads look good in green. Peanut butter needs jelly. What goes with making peace? Justice and Joy.

Peace is more than the absence of war. People can be put down and oppressed into a kind of silence that rulers mistakenly call peace. As a state of being, peace isn't possible unless justice is served and joy is present.

As a peacemaker, you observe strained silences among coworkers and residents, knowing justice is not being served. Management can play favorites, announce policies without asking for ideas, and change lives by thoughtlessly swapping roommates or scheduled work hours. Living and working where one's voice isn't heard is not peaceful. Justice and joy are not present. What is a peacemaker to do?

Marian Wright Edelman asked the same question of the world in a speech at Howard University Chapel in Washington, D.C.:

> The twentieth century has been characterized by stunning scientific and technological progress: we split the atom, pierced space, walked on the moon, landed on Mars and broke the genetic code. Instant communication has led to an information explosion and daily money trading in the trillions...But something today is missing from these stunning achievements. UNICEF reports that more babies are born into poverty than ever before. Over 840 million of our brothers and sisters in the world are malnourished, including 160 million children, who still die at a rate of 40,000 a day.

> Just three of America's richest people have wealth that totals $155 billion, equivalent to the gross national product of the 32 least economically developed countries in the world, containing 800 million people...How can our boastfully wealthy nation, which leads the world in millionaires and billionaires, look itself in the mirror each morning, when one in five, or 13.5 million, children are still poor?

President of the Children's Defense Fund, Mrs. Edelman spoke at the opening of the People's Campaign for Nonviolence. She detailed the glorification of violence, and wondered when we will stand up against the culture of death:

> Since 1979 we have lost over 80,000 American children to gunfire. That's 20,000 more children dead to guns than we lost in the Vietnam War. What has happened to us that the killing of children by guns has become routine: one every two hours?

> It is all interrelated. The United States leads the world in military expenditures and exports: we spend more in one week on the military than we spend annually on Head Start. Something is wrong with the values of a nation that would rather spend $20,000 or $30,000 to lock up a child after getting into trouble, than give them a head start.

As peacemaking caregivers, let's be inspired by Mrs. Edelman's encouragement to work together to create peace with justice and joy.

TODAY: *Speak up for justice and joy.*

When I was a young teenager, my mother took me on peace marches. By train, car and bus, we traveled around the Midwest and East coast on weekends, joining others calling for an end to war. The protesters' faces became my personal reference point, my definition of a peacemaker.

Returning to eighth grade homeroom on Monday morning, kids would talk about what they did on the weekend. "My mom and I went to Washington, D.C. for a peace march." Sure.

Later in life, after spending hours in nursing homes and residential care homes, I began to see that being a peacemaker could mean more than marching for peace. Observing the compassion of caregivers, I realized peacemakers could actually make peace. For some caregivers, this awareness feels like a daunting assignment, almost more than they can handle.

Jeanne is a highly conscientious nurse, a good-hearted woman with a tendency to take on the weight of the world. Sometimes her expression is pretty grim, revealing a heavy heart. When Tanyanne sees her in this mood, she gives her a hug and says, "Lighten up, Girlfriend! You're beautiful when you lighten up." Per their agreement, Jeanne thanks Tanyanne for reminding her that she is taking herself and others too seriously.

Jeanne sent Tanyanne a card that read:

> I love you for putting your hand into my heaped-up heart and passing over all the foolish and frivolous and weak things, and drawing out into the Light all the beautiful, radiant belongings that no one else had looked quite far enough to find.

Find a peace partner at work, someone who will help you be gentle with yourself and others. When making peace, keep it light.

TODAY: *Find a peace partner.*

Romanticizing the comforts of aging in one's home is an understandable fantasy. Newspapers tell us that institutions are big, bleak boxes on the outside of town, full of sick strangers. Who wouldn't want to be at home?

The reality is that more abuse, neglect and exploitation of the elderly occur at the hands of family members than at those of strangers. So much for fearing institutional care!

"People requiring care at home deal with a variety of people, ranging from a home care coordinator, to the home support staff that meets the person's specific needs," writes Teresa Stacey, a professional home care worker in Calgary, Alberta, Canada.

She continues:

> One also has to remember that there are many different needs, as well as many different personalities in the community. The in-home support agency carefully tries to maintain a balance, meeting each of these needs, with little disruption to the person in the home. A consistent care plan and caregiver are priorities for each client. We try to minimize the fear of new people, as constant change can be very stressful to a home client. Communication between the workers, agency and family members creates harmony in what could be a stressful time for families.

TODAY: *Communicate to create harmony.*

The Legend of Nicola

There were a people from the south who left their home-land on account of a quarrel that started when two men argued over what caused the soft, whistling, whisper-like sound made by a flock of geese in flight. One man said the noise came from their wings flapping, the other that it came from their bills. People took sides.

Finally the issue was submitted to the chief, who decided the noise was made through the bill. This angered the man who thought it was caused by the wings. A council was called to consider the question and it was decided for the bill. The man still believed in the wing. His relatives and friends got angry with chief and the council too, so they packed up and left the tribe. The Nicola became the "lost" band of the Wasco-Wishram, Chinookan living around the Dalles neighborhood of the Columbia River.

To be human is to disagree. Discord may hold all involved by the throat and seem silly to observers. What we fight about reveals the contents of our hearts. When something we value is threatened, we fight. The legend of the Nicola tribe is particularly beautiful. Awareness of nature was essential to the Indians' survival and happiness. We should not be surprised how an argument about one of nature's mysteries factors into the history of the Nicola people.

In my childhood, cowboys and Indians were important. Not only did the kids in the neighborhood play these parts in long afternoon games, but the few television programs we watched were Westerns. I learned early and often that the Red Man was violent and bloodthirsty. Only the Lone Ranger's Indian sidekick, Tonto, was a peacemaker. Even the word "sidekick" taught me the Indian was secondary. He was not a partner or equal to the white man.

In 1998, Ester Vanderwoude, a CNA from California, taught me a life lesson. While conducting a leadership workshop for extraordinary nursing assistants, I said that being out front had its hazards. "Remember, the pioneers are the ones with the arrows in their backs," I joked, without any real thought or reflection.

"Hey!" is all Ester had to say. Her face said the rest.

What a moment of revelation! I was simply parroting the myths of my childhood. What did I know about how Native Americans lived or conducted themselves? Later I apologized, and I thanked Ester. I also promised myself I would get educated, and learn about the Red Man's culture.

On July 3, 10, 15, 22 and 27 I have shared some of what I learned. A Smithsonian exhibit depicting the way Indians lived in total harmony with their environment also had a great influence on me, especially when I considered where the museum had acquired all the authentic clothing, tools and other gear. Stolen, I expect.

Like other peoples who have lived close to the land, the Indians of North America were peaceful nations with a true reverence for life. Conflicts were worked out in ways that didn't require extermination. We can learn a great deal from their ways.

TODAY: *Join the band of peacemakers.*

(Reprinted from *Mourning Dove: A Salishan Autobiography* edited by Jay Miller by permission of the University of Nebraska Press. Copyright © 1990 by the University of Nebraska Press.)

August: Blessed are those who have been persecuted for the cause of right, theirs is the kingdom of heaven.

In this last Beatitude, the faithful are promised the kingdom of heaven, the same blessing granted to the poor in spirit in the first Beatitude.

In the January Beatitude, we are taught that for being good humble souls, heaven is ours. And here, at the end of the string of blessings, we are promised heaven again, this time because we have endured criticism for living right.

Living a life committed to world health and well-being is a bold act. Unwilling to overlook poor quality or shoddy standards, caregivers speak up to intimidating supervisors and corporate giants. Calling for adequate time and resources, caregivers have been written up, dressed down and unfairly terminated by employers who don't share their sense of justice.

Caregivers are also insulted, misunderstood and harassed by resident family members, state inspectors, the media and, on occasion, their own families and friends. To be falsely accused is painful, particularly when one only seeks to do what is right.

Again and again, mature caregivers are reminded not to look to the world for affirmation or praise. In fact, far from being treated with high regard and being paid according to your extraordinary worth, you may be falsely judged and cast off in favor of less principled workers. At such times we are to hold our heads high and know we are loved for our brave hearts. Persecution drives us deeper into our life of faith, into the kingdom of heaven. Sure, it may seem easier to back away and remain silent. But how do we want to be known— as weak pushovers or as upholders of good?

The world's approval is not the prize. Caregivers answer to a higher power, one that commands us to love one another as we love ourselves.

Because I knew all parties, I knew the truth. Few of us enjoy this luxury when rumors fly, making it impossible to know what is real and what is made up.

Katie was looking for a new job. After twenty years in government she was ready for a complete change, and decided long-term care was the answer. "I don't want a lot of work to take home at night," she confided. "I need to be close to people but still leave the job at the end of the day."

Being activities director in a small nursing home was a perfect fit. Six months later, after she had been promoted to director of admissions and social services while still overseeing the activities department, Katie called me. "I came here to slow down, and they keep asking me to take on more." A bright, self-motivated employee, she had gained the owner's confidence. Promotion was inevitable.

Meanwhile, others at the facility called, "Katie has a Napoleon Complex! She wants to take over the world. Nobody's job is safe; that woman is determined to run this place!"

When the administrator left and Katie was asked to study for her nursing home administrator's license, the gossips went wild.

"Well, so much for taking a break," Katie joked, accepting the responsibility of managing the facility. A strong and gentle woman, she focused on being close with residents and staff, true to her original call to the work. As for the gossip and persecution, she rose above it with love.

TODAY: *Rise above gossip.*

When a certain associate of my husband's visits, she always begins bashing men. Dee Dee is pretty angry with men, and pretty funny in her anger. I swear her nasty humor is contagious, and before long, we are both picking on my bewildered husband.

Like breadcrumbs in the meatloaf, people can easily take on the flavor of an overpowering presence. I find my "hamburger helper attitude" really shows up when I'm around depressed people. Before long, I join their chorus of moans about why the weather stinks, the economy is worse and diets don't work.

The victim of a mood pickpocket, I'm robbed of my spirit. Wait a minute! I love my husband, and life, too. Why have I surrendered to these negative forces?

Misery loves company. Unhappy people want to be the lowest common denominator, subconsciously craving the company of other criers. And nothing is more comforting than dragging a positive soul down.

At home and in the workplace, avoid detours off the high road. Invite the sad and mad to join your sunny walk. As we age, we learn that we attract our own definitions of the world. If we imagine all men are stinkers, that's who asks us out.

TODAY: *Define your life.*

"Why" questions torture us.

Why did she say she was going to meet with all of us in the first month? Why did she say we would get raises? Why did she say she would have staff meetings? She didn't do any of that!

Employees at a West Coast facility were angry and hurt by the new administrator's broken promises. Brought in to clean up a big mess, Mrs. Dale had grand plans. She wanted to meet with staff and listen to concerns. Changes would be made. Improvements were guaranteed.

Three months into her administration, Mrs. Dale hadn't gotten one balloon off the ground. Employees all told their own versions of the same story: "How Mrs. Dale Let Me Down."

The less confident staff doubted themselves, dwelling on why Mrs. Dale had canceled their appointments.

Like an owl perched high on the edge of the woods, Jill said:

> I've been through this before. People come to a place like gangbusters, ready to change the world. They get in that office on the phone, and never come out. I'm not saying it doesn't hurt to be let down. But why obsess over it? I stay away from 'why' questions. I ask instead what I can learn from what I have observed. What do I need to let go of? You can feel persecuted or even persecute yourself, but that's pointless. We have to move on.

Regardless of disappointments, our spirits need not be damaged. Consider these events a stone in your shoe. Shake it out and keep on moving, doing what you do so well.

TODAY: *Shake off letdowns.*

Career nursing assistant Jeanne Dimick of Tomah, Wisconsin (the cranberry center of the universe), decided to take a stand. What she was reading in the papers and seeing on television about nursing homes simply did not mirror her 25 years of experience.

Promoting a poor image of nursing homes, the media "criticizes caregivers without recognizing the work we do," Jeanne wrote in a letter to reporters. She continued:

> Without us, what would happen to our elderly? The public needs to know the true role of the caregiver. It is not just the skill of being a CNA; it is loyalty, commitment and devotion to the aging. Most of us have dedicated our lives to quality care; we choose our profession because we are caring people.

> The work is hard and frustrating, but we get so much in return, this is a privilege. Our job is a rewarding one. You need to be a special person to bring happiness to another person's day.

Sitting back and complaining about media coverage doesn't change anything, and actually allows the erosion of truth to continue. As the late First Lady and humanitarian Eleanor Roosevelt said, "No one can hurt you without your consent."

Jeanne Dimeck refuses to consent. "Come to visit us sometime," Jeanne wrote, "the welcome sign is always hanging. Come observe the love, care and concern that exist in nursing homes. I know there are lots of positive things to say about nursing homes—I work in one."

TODAY: *Take a stand.*

Compassion is not something reserved for the starving children of Africa or the political prisoners of China. Compassion is a daily, ongoing practice.

Bob was being teased by other nurses for his "weird handwriting."

"We can hardly read those smeared streaks!" they'd say. "Chicken scratchings would be clearer."

Bob was new on the job and had not shared his struggle to become a nurse. Raised by this grandmother, who was a nurse, Bob decided when he was a little boy that he wanted to follow in Gran's footsteps. But since he was dyslexic, achieving that dream caused many sleepless nights.

"I had special tutors and it took me almost three years," Bob told Susie, the staff developer. Susie was the compassionate listener he needed. "I've learned a lot about learning disabilities. Do you know that left-handed people have a much higher incidence of dyslexia, migraines, allergies, and autoimmune disorders like arthritis? I'm left-handed and my hand slides across the ink when I write."

Bob worked with Susie on improving his notes, using a special smear-proof pen. Susie also did an in-service without naming names on tolerance and differences for the nursing staff.

Thanks to his grandmother's powerful belief in him, Bob was licensed as a practical nurse. "Gran read that left-handed people have talent in math, and wouldn't you know it, that was my best subject!"

"Some things may take me longer to do than other people, but I'm going to make it! I love being a nurse," Bob said.

TODAY: *Find compassionate support.*

I had known this adorable director of nursing for at least 10 years. A sweet sprite of a woman, this was her last job. "I can't believe retirement is nearly here," Nora said, "I'm not sure I'm ready."

A nurse for 40 years, Nora's mixed feelings were completely understandable. Retirement resembled a divorce or death, as nursing was such a part of her life.

Back at the facility, the snotty jokes about Nora's old ways accelerated as her retirement date approached. "She still wears a cap to meetings with the state! What a dinosaur!"

Tammy was in her third year of nursing, a baby by Nora's standards. A reserved young woman, Tammy shied away from conflict. All the same, she couldn't sit and listen to other nurses mock their retiring director. In the midst of the meanness, Tammy quietly mixed in words and acts of kindness. Working with others, she planned a surprise retirement coffee hour, asking Nora's family to provide some old photos of Nora's nursing career to decorate the room.

Hearing how Tammy rose above these nasty conditions, I was reminded of the fact that good perfume is made from contrary-smelling substances, like skunk oil and flowers. Because of the way contraries interact with one another, the elements that make up the scent aren't easy to pick out; it is neither one thing nor the other. As the fragrant rose, Tammy blended in with the skunks, and created a beautiful finale to Nora's extraordinary lifetime of service.

Feel like a shy rose in a garden of skunks? Be brave! Your love will not be overpowered.

TODAY: *Be brave.*

"If I have to go to a nursing home, shoot me!"

"I'll float out to sea on an iceberg before I go into that place."

Working in health care, we hear these dramatic statements from people who believe the media's horror stories. Too busy working, few caregivers take time to write or tell wonderful stories of care, so the public remains frightened and uneducated about nursing home life.

Some caregivers, bombarded with bad news, begin to hide, believing they are unworthy losers. The great pacifist leader Mahatma Gandhi, who was also slandered in the press, once said, "They cannot take away our self-respect if we do not give it to them."

Far from giving away their self-respect, the employees of Little Flower Manor in Scranton, Pennsylvania proudly share their mission statement with the community.

"Our mission is to promote the Christian mission of healing care, by assuring...quality of life based on respect, care and compassion for the whole person." Further, the quality of life at Little Flower is, "surrounded by a spirit that fosters human dignity and self-esteem within a homelike environment committed to the sanctity of life."

TODAY: *Proudly share your mission.*

During a workshop on religious tolerance in Belfast, Northern Ireland, a young teacher asked a question of the multi-faith panel:

> I am a Buddhist, and I teach in a Christian elementary school in Japan. The families are Christians from other nations, living in Japan. I have been trying to get to know my students' parents, but nothing seems to work. Do you have any ideas?

The panelists asked her to describe what wasn't working. She answered:

> Well, I have held open houses at all different times of day, hoping to get the parents to drop in and talk. I've been told they don't like me because I'm a Buddhist. But we share their children, so I feel it is important we communicate. I don't know what to do.

The moderator asked an Anglican bishop seated on the panel what he would recommend. He replied dryly, "Sounds like she needs to convert the Christians to Christianity."

How many times have you thought the same thing, having been treated poorly by an individual wearing a big cross around his or her neck? I have always gotten a kick out of church parking lot behavior. Having just encountered one hour of Christian instruction, it is amazing how few drivers let another car exit before them.

As loving caregivers with a deep sense of purpose you are role models. People are watching.

TODAY: *Practice what you preach.*

Barbara has been a nursing assistant more than half her life. All but one of her 31 years of caring for others has been in the same northern Indiana nursing home. Queen Barbara is what they call her. But what interrupted Barbara's extraordinary record of service during her 29 th year as a professional caregiver?

"I was suspended for 90 days," Barbara said, her eyes revealing a broken heart. Certified to dispense medications, Barbara was passing pills on the evening shift with an LPN when the only other nurse in the building went home sick. "My nurse went to the other wing to do medications and she told another CNA on my wing, who wasn't certified to handle medications, to help me dispense pills. She was studying to become a Qualified Medication Assistant, or QMA, but she wasn't one yet."

The next morning, an angry administrator informed Barbara she should not have worked with the CNA. "Come back in 90 days and we'll discuss your employment." No appeal process was described or offered.

Exactly 90 days later, Barbara returned, only to be told she would not be considered for re-employment for a full year.

"These residents are my babies," Barbara said. "And this job is my life. I can tell you the very day I started in Chicago, Illinois, on August 15, 1967. That woman didn't even let me tell my side of the story. She said it was a serious violation of safety rules and I was escorted from the building."

Barbara found immediate employment in a neighboring facility, but 365 days later, with her head high, she returned: "Home, where I belong."

Amazingly, the administrator had been replaced, and Barbara was welcomed back. Residents and coworkers rejoiced.

"I would never hurt these people. I love them," Barbara says, glad she is back where she belongs.

TODAY: *Hold your head high.*

Buddhist tradition teaches that after the Lord Buddha died, five hundred of his disciples met to recall the truths they had received from their beloved teacher during the forty-five years of his ministry.

With the teacher no longer among them and no written texts, the monks prepared talks on basic themes. A compilation of 300 talks was assembled and called the Dhammapada. Put in verse form, the couplets contrast the vanity of hypocrisy, false pride, heedlessness, and selfish desire with the virtues of truthfulness, modesty and vigilance.

Marguerite Reynolds, a Florida nursing assistant, sent me this verse from the Dhammapada: "Pay no attention to harsh words uttered by others. Do not be concerned with what others have or have not. Observe your own actions or inactions."

Just 26 words to live by. Where is it practiced?

Definitely on the night shift in nursing homes. Have you noticed the different personality of each shift? Here are some generalizations I've collected. On days, staff can get pretty worked up. The evening shift is full of laid-back staff. But nights—that's where the happy people seem to be.

What causes this phenomenon? I've heard some neat theories, including that as the number of department heads decline, the mood of the staff improves. Also, that as the pace of the day winds down, the spirits rise.

Whatever the cause, the important distinction here is that shifts do have personalities that influence moods and behavior. Being aware of the environmental tone, we can protect ourselves. We can learn to follow Marguerite's Dhammapada advice.

TODAY: *Observe.*

A colleague sent me an advertisement that appeared in a Missouri newspaper: "Wanted, dead or alive! LPNs, CNAs or non-certified assistants." In smaller print it says, "Really, live people are what we are looking for!"

We ranted and raved to one another, wondering in particular how people who live and work at the facility would regard the ad.

"Can you imagine being a family member of a resident, and seeing how desperate the facility is for staff?"

"What about being an employee and realizing warm bodies are the standard?"

The human animal makes mistakes. Stupid mistakes. Big, stupid mistakes that can hurt others. When you witness a mistake, remember to drink an extra cup of Instant Tolerance before you speak.

For employees working in facilities that place demeaning, ignorant advertising, consider getting a group together and offering to help write the next ads. What should be said to potential employees? How would you invite someone to join your team? Be tolerant, strong and creative to make lasting change.

TODAY: *Be tolerant, strong and creative.*

Responsible for close to 20 nursing homes in a western state, Mary worked 90 hours a week and loved it. Single, she brought her dog to work so she didn't have to rush home at night. Known for ironclad goals and a steel spine, Mary achieved what she set out to do. More like a Marine than the petite accountant she was, Mary demanded a great deal of the regional office staff. They loved her, and were terrified to fail her.

Among the gag gifts Mary received at her office birthday party was a homemade electric collar. "They know I want to zap some staff into higher performance, so they made me this!" she laughed. Would the administrators Mary wants to "zap" find the collar funny? If not, the gift should be tossed.

The collar reminded me of another inappropriate office decoration I saw in a catalogue: "Barrels of fun! Hand-painted jars for spare change, candy, paper clips or jewelry. Kiln fired, hand-glazed, hand-dipped ceramic."

Sound lovely? Not with the message "Hand lettered with 'Ashes of Problem Employees.' $15.95."

With the staffing challenges in long-term care, even in jest the presence of such joke items is extremely hazardous to everyone's health. High-quality caregivers have a great sense of humor that doesn't get activated at the expense of others. Be careful about bringing these kinds of novelties to work. Think about how every single party will react. Then think one more time. Do no harm.

TODAY: *Be a careful joker.*

Quarrel with the math, but consider the basic idea. If we estimate each nursing home resident in the nation's 17,000 facilities receives one ounce more food than s/he can eat at each meal, we throw away more than 212 tons of food a day! (One hundred residents per facility, served three meals daily.)

I believe we throw away more food because government-required portion sizes are simply too big for the average frail elder. How many 110-pound, 86-year-old ladies do you know who eat an 8-ounce pork chop for lunch? Convinced facilities would underfeed residents, regulators specify meal requirements, right down to how many canned peach slices shall garnish a scoop of cottage cheese.

Let's take my math one step further and estimate wasted food costs five cents an ounce. Thrown out in one year? $124 million worth of food. (6.8 million ounces multiplied by 5 cents multiplied by 365 days) I imagine every reader has some ideas for how that money could be spent.

Determined caregivers, armed with passion and facts, are the only individuals who can end this waste. Regulators and lawmakers do not work in healthcare facilities; they do not know what would work better than government attempts at standardizing care.

Carole Bouchard, a home care aide in Calgary, Alberta, proposes caregivers slip on a second hat, that of activist, in order to improve the quality of home care in Canada:

> We first need to lobby government officials for increased cash flow for wages and training for front-line workers. We need to have alternate living arrangements for clients whose families cannot emotionally deal with their illness in the family home. We need increased funding for hospice care outside the home, for sometimes the home is not the best place to be when a loved one is dying. We need small, intimate, community-based nursing homes—maybe our old empty community schools could be renovated—to keep our seniors in

their home communities. We also need to ensure that nursing homes increase the level of privacy for individuals—one room to one person with a window that opens. And we need to lessen the staff-patient ratio in hospitals and nursing homes.

TODAY: *Be an activist.*

From the pages of a Michigan activities director's journal:

Just had our annual survey this week. Not too bad, but not completely fair, like usual. I got a citation for not following the care plan for one of my residents, which is totally not true.

The surveyor stopped me in the hall and asked me about a resident, and of course, I am supposed to instantly know all health problems of all 220-plus residents on demand. This resident was on a unit that I assigned to someone else, so I didn't know her personally. Surveys are VERY disheartening to those of us who work at our best each and every day.

Unfortunately, surveys are more than feedback. I have known excellent people to lose their jobs over bad surveys. And the monetary damages have driven several providers right out of business in the area.

We have a survey team that is notorious for being rude. One of our CNAs of 20 years nearly quit over the way she was treated by a surveyor last year. Praise God, she stayed and became a voice at our state's healthcare association's annual legislation day.

Why do extraordinary caregivers allow themselves to be set up and then devastated by surveys? I cringe at the idea of anything similar occurring in our personal lives. What would they say about the nights we have popcorn and wine for dinner? Or the winter weekends I stay in my PJs for two days! I have watched excellent, dedicated DONs fall apart or quit after at a bad survey, taking the state's assessment of their performance literally.

The activities director's journal entry is a sobering reminder that the world of long-term care is truly in need of major realignment. Can nursing homes successfully serve elders in this regulatory environment? When it becomes commonplace for state survey teams to issue 60 or more pages of deficiencies for an annual survey, it seems clear the government isn't doing a good job either.

May the last tear over a nursing home survey be shed. Let's move on to creating a system for assuring quality that works. In the meantime, remember you are more than a survey.

TODAY: *Keep the survey in its place.*

As a former newspaper reporter and editor, I believe the secret to successful media relations is in the relations.

If you want the attention of your local paper or television station, first give them attention. Rather than calling blindly and talking to whomever answers the phone in the newsroom, create a strategy.

1. Pull a group of volunteers together to watch the local evening news and/or read the local paper for a set period of time (one to three weeks.)

2. Ask the group to track the stories/features they liked, noting the reporter's name.

3. With data collected, compare notes. Identify the overall favorite reporter(s).

4. Determine the best time to visit the newsroom. Pay attention to deadlines. If the paper is distributed in the afternoon, the deadline is probably late morning. Don't call and ask for an appointment with your favorite reporter when s/he is madly trying to meet a deadline.

5. Have a few members of your group meet with the reporter. Share your appreciation of specific stories or articles s/he wrote: "We loved the piece you did on the new teen drop-in center! Based on the work you've been doing, we think we have some stories in our facility that you might like to write."

6. Provide the reporter with a few ideas to tease their interest, such as a paragraph on your alert resident who flew with Amelia Earhart or learned to drive in Winston Churchill's car. Interest him/her in coming to your facility, and fishing for unusual stories.

7. Ask the reporter how s/he would like to be contacted. Can you call them once a month with story ideas? Would they prefer a personal visit to their newsroom? Explain your desire to see good news of your facility in the paper, to improve staff morale and remind residents they are worthy members of the community at large.

8. Invite your favorite reporter to a special luncheon or other activity, so s/he can become acquainted with the spirit of the facility. Perhaps they would like to speak at a staff meeting or volunteer recognition banquet? Consider giving them an award later in the year for the positive press they have given you.

Start with the smallest newspaper, such as the weekly shoppers' guide. Most of these little publications are hungry for copy and will welcome your ideas, photos and articles.

Enjoy your pursuit! Your desire to provide readers and viewers with good, positive news is a noble and healthy goal. You will succeed.

TODAY: *Provide good news.*

Public indifference to the needs of others is not unique to our times. Throughout history, the masses have had to be challenged to accept their civic duty. A description of almshouses, this was written in the 1850s by a committee of the New York legislature:

> Our citizens manifest so little interest in the condition even of those in their immediate neighborhood. Individuals who take great interest in human suffering whenever it is brought to their notice, never visit them, and are entirely uninformed, that in a country house almost at their own doors, may be found the lunatic suffering for years in a dark and suffocating cell, in summer, and almost freezing the winter—where a score of children are poorly fed, poorly clothed and quite untaught—where the poor idiot is half starved and beaten with rods because he is too dull to do his master's bidding—where the aged mother is lying in perhaps her last sickness, unattended by a physician, and with no one to minister to her wants—where the lunatic, too, a woman, is made to feel the lash in the hands of a brutal underkeeper—yet these are all to be found; they all exist in our state.

Homes for the poor, almshouses were also known as "social cemeteries" and "living tombs." Dedicated men and women went to work every day in these institutions, cooking meals, washing clothing, cleaning floors, serving the residents.

Surely misunderstood by the community, underpaid and even risking their health, good-hearted individuals stepped forward when families could no longer care. And as for the brutal underkeeper, for the sake of justice, let's hope he was challenged.

TODAY: *Challenge.*

(Reprinted with the permission of The Free Press, a Division of Simon & Schuster, Inc., from *From Poor Law to Welfare State: A History of Social Welfare in America* by Walter I. Trattner. Copyright © 1974, 1979, 1984, 1989 by The Free Press. Copyright © 1994, 1998 by Walter I. Trattner.)

Tina had not received a raise in two years. Business was not good, management told the front-line caregivers. "Wait until next January; we may be able to do something then."

A single mother raising three children, Tina knew more than she wanted to about creative financing and where all the dented-can stores were in town. When January rolled around, she was the first associate at the administrator's door.

"I wondered if I will get a raise this year? You told us maybe in January."

"Stand up on that chair," the administrator directed. Confused, Tina did so.

"That is as much of a raise as you're going to get."

On behalf of the families and residents of nursing homes, to all those caregivers who have been insulted, degraded and demeaned, please know how much you are appreciated. Yes, your day will come, when the culture awakens to your value and compensates you fully. Bless you for working in sometimes unfriendly conditions. You surely have a place waiting in the kingdom of heaven.

TODAY: *Know you are valued.*

My robust parents are in their seventies, blessed with full heads of thick white hair. Chronologically, they are labeled senior citizens. To those who know them, Roger and Kay Greeley are still heat-seeking missiles, heading for action.

Talking with others in their age bracket, they discovered an annoying common experience: being ignored when transacting business. A retired minister and a retired teacher, my parents have both always commanded the attention of individuals and groups. Never brushed off earlier in life, they believe such treatment can be attributed to one factor: they look old.

Tasteless greeting cards aimed at older people are also offensive. Reaching great age milestones isn't a grand achievement, it is cause of cruel humor about deteriorating mental and physical prowess.

Accepting this crude humor, we travel one step closer to an even more dangerous expression of age discrimination, the belief that elders are burdens to themselves and others. If society insists the young and old are burdens, is life One Big Burden? Each of us needs plenty from others: responses, reactions, support, acknowledgement and conversation. If the old are a burden, then we all are a burden.

Caregivers who know the joys of serving others are obligated to set the record straight. Human beings are not burdens. Human beings are our passports to heaven.

TODAY: *Celebrate age.*

I receive this note from a wonderful aide who gives her life to her work. I hurt knowing she has been hurt.

> Why do people we work with like to play games with other people's jobs and lives? I have tried to work with different people but these nurses are the hardest I've ever dealt with. (Yes I said my prayers tonight.) None of the CNAs want to work with two of the LPNs on 3-11. Tonight I was ready to quit my job. Why do LPNs feel they are better than CNAs? We work very hard. Take the titles away and you should have people who care.

Unfortunately, the nursing home has inherited the bad habits of its older sister, the hospital. Historically, doctors have not regarded nurses as peers. Treated as stupid and second class, the nurse passes disrespect on to those who report to her.

Staff should not take such persecution personally, as it is not about them, but about the pecking order. Some people only stand tall and feel good about themselves when they believe someone is below them.

Responding with healthy anger is appropriate. The function of anger is similar to the function of a fever: it helps to burn out unwanted, inharmonious elements and restore balance and well-being.

> Anger is not an accurate evaluation or judgment of who a person actually is. Anger is merely our own feelings communicating with us, telling us more about ourselves than about that other person. It is the beginning of greater clarity and discrimination, so that we can live our passion with integrity, develop our inner power, and become capable of acting assertively, rather than aggressively, on behalf of what we cherish.

TODAY: *Develop inner power.*

(From the book *The Awakened Heart.* Revised edition copyright © 1997 by John Robbins and Ann Mortifee. Reprinted with permission of H J Kramer/New World Library, Novato, CA. www.newworldlibrary.com or 800-972-6657 ext. 52.)

At five my son knew words and world conditions that did not enter my consciousness until I was in my twenties: AIDS, handgun violence, pollution and global warming. Today, in his early twenties, he is worried about stock market vulnerabilities and Third World countries owning nuclear warheads. Nearly 50, I only recently began considering these latest threats to world stability.

The questioning of older generations is an expected right of passage. Most adolescents find their parents incredibly dense, an attitude that kicks off teenage rebellion. But in this millennium, young people may have a legitimate claim against their predecessors.

The planet is in trouble, and it looks like the kids are going to have to fix it. Persecuted by a careless past, they have every right to rail against our poor stewardship.

Farmers tell us it can take four generations to restore soil that has been hurt by one generation. In the healthcare setting, healthy growth can be delayed by similar poor management.

Homes that have been repeatedly sold or experienced frequent turnover of administration cannot produce a good crop of caregivers. Like the farmer's depleted land, these facilities haven't got what it takes to yield bounty. Working in barren buildings stripped of their vitality, quality caregivers must take one day at a time, looking for small successes and incremental change. Gradually, the necessary ingredients come together, and suddenly it is clear life is improving. No longer a victim of history, the new group of healers begins to plant a patch of heaven.

TODAY: *Plant a patch of heaven.*

Admitting a loved one is abusive has to be one of life's most difficult assignments. Deep within the human seed is an inborn certainty that families care.

Lenore had been with Bud since she was an 18-year-old headed for nursing school and he was nearly 40. A handsome contractor, Bud picked Lenore out of the crowd and neither looked back—until Lenore turned 45 and Bud was in his late sixties. Life was no longer weekends of dancing and drinking. Owner of a multi-million-dollar regional home health agency, Lenore was a successful and attractive businesswoman. Bud's lifestyle had robbed him of his health and rugged good looks. He began to imagine that every man who spoke to Lenore wanted her, and accused her of egging them on.

Around this same time, Lenore began to receive threatening calls at work. The gruff voice warned her she was being watched, "through the scope of a Winchester rifle." Confiding in her colleagues, Lenore was frightened and baffled: "Who could be doing this to me?"

Everyone but Lenore had their suspicions, particularly after hearing her husband's screaming fits in the parking lot. "He's just not feeling good, he would never hurt me!" Lenore insisted angrily. Feeling betrayed by her secretary's suggestion that Bud was the culprit, Lenore fired her. Other friendships began to go sour as Lenore turned on anyone who said Bud was being abusive.

At her brother's insistence, Lenore had the police monitor phone calls at work. The death threats were traced to her husband. Humiliated, Lenore went to friends and family in tears and apologized.

She saw she had abused anyone who had dared mention Bud's abusiveness. Gradually, Lenore restored the relationships she had destroyed. Her secretary had the grace to return to work, telling Lorraine she would "do it all again if she had to."

Today: *Stand up to abuse.*

Mark works several jobs as a nursing assistant. "Believe me, I don't want to be driving all over town, trying to remember where I'm supposed to be on what day," he said. "But they won't give me any overtime at Forestdale, so I have to work for the agency and do private duty."

A married father of two, Mark feels he was born to be a CNA. Still, when it's time to pay the bills, the family questions Mark's career choice. "Like it's not tough enough as it is, what really hurts is when Forestdale calls and asks if I can work on my day off or do a double shift, and they get mad because I have to go to my other job!" Having worked with this arrangement for five years, Mark decided long ago it did no good to remind the director of nursing that the facility's no-overtime policies give him no choice.

"She'll say it isn't her decision, that she would love to pay overtime," Mark said. "I just say I'm sorry I can't come in."

When we were little kids, our mothers told us life isn't fair. Why must we continue to receive reminders?

The financing of health care is the real villain here. At some point, we'll create a way to pay caregivers a living wage. Blessed be the caregivers, persecuted for hanging in there! Your residents and their families sing your praises.

TODAY: *Create your schedule.*

As a long-term care ombudsman, I resolved complaints, free and confidentially, for residents of Vermont nursing homes and residential care homes. My contact with people was intimate and intense.

Called by the resident or other interested party, sometimes anonymously, I would investigate the complaint and make recommendations. All of my cases were interesting, simply because they were about people's lives.

Some lives, though, were absolutely fascinating. Marcella Foss led the fascinating category. Her initial call was about the food served at a small care home where she and her husband, both vegetarians, lived. The owners of the home were not living up to the Fosses' expectations, and Marcella wanted me to get the meals upgraded.

I don't recall Mr. Foss ever speaking, though he probably offered me a greeting when we met. He really didn't need to, as Marcella was so efficient. Could she describe what she would like for meals?

Marcella Foss pulled a spiral notebook from the center of a bookshelf of notebooks that was about two and a half feet long. "In 1979, we lived at the Canterbury Inn. While their laundry facilities were utterly below grade, the redeeming factor was clearly the kitchen. Wasn't it, Wendell?" He nodded.

"What are you reading from?" I asked.

"My log from that year," Mrs. Foss said with some pride. Though I had hoped to keep the appointment to an hour, I couldn't resist asking about the other spiral notebooks that filled the shelf. Mrs. Foss had logs itemizing her dissatisfaction with life going back to their first year of marriage! I had never met a professional complainer before.

This past year, Maxine Burns, the daughter of a deceased nursing home resident, contacted me about the "barbaric neglect" her mother suffered in a nursing home. As we communicated, I recalled Marcella Foss.

Neither woman could be satisfied. To whatever suggestion I offered, these women could dish out five reasons why I was naïve, nuts and misinformed.

Maxine told me she would remain angry the rest of her life for how her mother had suffered in a nursing home. I wrote her a note:

> I am truly sorry that the pain you experienced is so great that you will be angry the rest of your life. As one woman to another, I feel sad about this, for you. Holding anger can cause physical and emotional illness. Forgiveness is powerful. It doesn't mean you think the other party was okay or right or fair. It just means you want to let go and move on.

When complaining, Maxine wrote me daily. I never heard from her again after I proposed she let go. Professional caregivers who face professional complainers know how to create respectful boundaries. Resolution is rarely the complainant's goal. Being aware of the nature of such interactions, harassment can be minimized.

TODAY: *Listen with boundaries.*

Persecution, like adversity, has its sweet uses. Clara Barton, founder of the American Red Cross, began her career nursing sick and wounded soldiers in the Civil War. In 1888, Barton recalled women's work in the Civil War and declared that because of it the American woman was "at least fifty years in advance of the normal position which continued peace...would have assigned."

American women of the pre-Civil War era were like their English counterparts, pampered in near-prisons of homes. Entertaining company and visiting the ill were about the only acceptable pastimes for the delicate female flower.

Women became involved in service during the war, and many never returned to the to solitude of domestic life. A brutal and bloody scar on the young nation, the Civil War launched some women on lifelong careers of service.

Out of tough circumstances great performances are born, as individuals rise to the occasion. Frightened when she first had to oversee the preparation of 300 meals daily after the head cook had a stroke, Bev's confidence grew over the ensuing months. To her own great surprise, Bev accepted the promotion and developed a reputation for preparing the best desserts in the city.

TODAY: *Grow from adversity.*

(Reprinted with the permission of The Free Press, a Division of Simon & Schuster, Inc., from *From Poor Law to Welfare State: A History of Social Welfare in America* by Walter I. Trattner. Copyright © 1974, 1979, 1984, 1989 by The Free Press. Copyright © 1994, 1998 by Walter I. Trattner.)

Lou, the staff developer, wanted to know why the nursing assistants had asked a company outsider, rather than him, about education benefits.

"We offer tuition reimbursement to full-time employees after they pass an approved nursing class," Lou said. "I don't understand why this question wasn't brought to me."

All of us carry demons—voices only we can hear—that make us doubt our talent and skills. Unless we had a childhood rich in encouragement, many caregivers are highly insecure about whether they could handle more responsibility.

"I haven't been to school for 15 years," Amy said. "I have no idea if I could even pass a class. They might think I'm too stupid to take one."

Haunted by low self-esteem, employees are too embarrassed to ask their supervisor about educational opportunities. When we're tortured by our insecurity, relief can come through opening up to a friend or admired associate at work. Dr. Timothy Conway writes:

> Many of us feel out of Love and incapable of living Love. Perhaps we are still shaken from a history of trauma, or resentful of abuse done to our persons, or ashamed of our past failures. Then let us be consoled and healed of our misery. Let us feel the warm caring, curative embrace of the Supreme Being through these women...If we only say 'yes' to the process, they can help release us from the pain of hurt, fear or guilt, by their harmonious resonance, vibrating us back into the feeling-current of Love.

Never underestimate the power of one loving, encouraging voice in your life. Instead of listening to the Inner Nag that doesn't think you can make it, treat yourself to the kind wisdom of a seasoned coworker.

TODAY: *Seek encouragement.*

Working on a project with the facility administrator meant I visited Hillshire Manor almost once a week for six months. A working professional 12 years of experience and a master's degree, I was confident on the job. Except when I entered Hillshire Manor and ran into Sandra, the director of nursing.

I was 38 years old and afraid of her! A bully of a woman, Sandra's greeting was usually, "What do you want?" or "Why are you here?" She was abrupt and humorless, and looked at me like I was about commit an illegal act.

As quickly as possible I would scoot into the office of Bill, the administrator. I couldn't fathom what it would be like to work in the facility daily with Sandra. On one visit I told Bill I was uncomfortable with Sandra's tough act. "I always feel I'm in trouble !" I said. He laughed and said Sandra wasn't so bad, but that she needed to be tough to keep staff in line.

Sandra left the job in a hurry, charged with embezzling patient funds. No wonder she suspected everyone else of crime! Employees came out of the woodwork upon her departure with their own horrid tales of Sandra's intimidation.

"Gentleness can only be expected from the strong," author Leo Roskin wrote. True leaders do not need to bully or mistrust. If you work in an environment of suspicion and tension, be careful to keep your sense of self-worth.

TODAY: *Hold tight to your self-confidence.*

Pearlie Mae joked:

> On my shift, the staff is in such a bad mood, nobody would say the glass was half-full. They wouldn't even say it was half-empty. They would probably say there wasn't even a glass there!

Workshop participants laughed, but they also nodded with sympathy. Anyone who has worked in health care for some time knows that facilities have mood swings and cycles, just like people.

"If I had had a dog at home, he would have been kicked," Pearlie Mae continued. "I finally talked to my pastor, because I was getting ready to quit."

The veteran aide of some 28 years shared her pastor's wise words:

> He reminded me about all of the people in the Bible who had suffered at the hands of others. Job was one. We talked about Jesus, and how he got in trouble just because he healed sick people on Sundays, talked to hookers and ate with tax collectors. I started to see my suffering differently, like it was my own cross.

A natural wit, with the full attention of the room, Pearlie Mae added:

> So I decided to just keep smiling. I'm working for one reason only: my little old men and women. I got to stay fit for them. As for the old sourpusses I work with, I told my pastor, as long as they don't crucify me, I guess I'm okay!

TODAY: *Keep smiling.*

"Sometimes, in the busyness of the day, we can forget to greet families and friends," wrote some CNAs from Southern California. "One family member told one of us that she felt very uncomfortable coming into our nursing home. So we wrote these Guidelines for Visitors."

1. The time of the visit is important. Come after 11 AM, or make an appointment so your loved one will be ready.

2. The length of the visit is entirely up to you—enjoy yourselves!

3. Have your visit anywhere you wish, except the dining room during meals. It is hard for us to assist our residents with a crowd present. If you do visit during a meal, ask us to set up a private table for you, and please make sure your loved one eats.

4. Yes! Please bring children, they are most welcome. Can you make sure they don't run?

5. If you bring food, please give it to your loved one after the meal and make sure it is OK for them to eat if they are on a special diet.

6. Ask for extra chairs if you need them, beverages or anything else to make your visit more enjoyable.

7. Feel free to ask CNAs for anything you need help with; we will help you find answers.

8. Share information with us about your loved one's habits, preferences, hobbies, interests. The better we know them, the better we can care for them.

9. If we are dressing your loved one in clothing you don't want him or her to wear, please take it with you. We use what we have.

Sometimes, the obvious is what we inadvertently ignore, and actually the most important part of the day. Can you sit down and create a protocol for visitors? A welcome visitor is less likely to complain or file a lawsuit.

TODAY: *Welcome visitors.*

Ancestry and ethnic background mean a great deal to some folks, often governing whether they consider someone worthy of friendship. History is full of persecution and discrimination based on religion, race or color.

Within the world of long-term care, a splinter element is criticizing those who work with or in healthcare facilities incorporated as profit-making businesses. According these self-appointed judges, only non-profit homes should be permitted to serve frail elders. All others are "corporate slime."

A young idealist in Florida, Rebecca Edwards heads up the Adopt a Grandperson Program introduced on these pages on March 1. "The program is a caring and creative solution to the loneliness and sense of abandonment a majority of Grandpersons experience living in healthcare residences," she says. "It also teaches valuable life lessons and provides opportunities for spiritual growth for volunteers, whom we call The Compassionates."

When Rebecca's mother, Sherry Ernst, founded AGP and the National CNA Friendship Society, she received insulting mail:

> You can either ally yourself with the profit-takers or with the people who they are victimizing—nursing home residents, their families, and their own rank-and-file employees. It's your choice.

> The corrupt, for-profit system needs to changed, not by (your) societies but by hell-raising, persistent complaining, undercover investigations using cameras and tape recorders, news media publicity, lawsuits, and public and noisy confrontation of legislators and enforcement agencies.

Ugh! I wonder what it would be like to live in nursing homes under such a state of siege? How can angry and invasive tactics be used in the name of good care?

To the woman or man in the bed, the facility's incorporated status means little or nothing. Some non-profit and for-prof it homes alike divert too many profits or, as labeled in the non-profit world, margins.

Listening to all parties involved with nursing home ministries, Sherry, Rebecca and their kindred spirits taste heaven. All other feedback is nonsense and can be ignored accordingly.

TODAY: *Taste heaven.*

State and federal governments periodically experiment with using more frequent unannounced inspections of health-care facilities to improve patient care. Who would want these quasi-police jobs, monitoring institutions on nights, weekends and holidays? An administrator once told me about receiving a surprise visit on New Year's Eve from a state survey nurse. "We had fired her two years ago for sleeping at work, and she came back to retaliate."

Harassment of this nature is tough to take. Meetings need to be organized for facility staff and state officials to identify common concerns for resident health. Facilities have more at stake here than government employees, so facilities must assume the lead role.

Gary R. Ilminen, an RN who works as a nurse consultant for Wisconsin Department of Health and Family Services, has been addressing this very matter for more than twenty years. Writing about government, health and environmental issues for local and regional newspapers and magazines, his major work is a *Consumer Guide to Long-term Care*.

> I firmly believe that national improvement cannot be achieved using HCFA's current belief that better inspections make better nursing homes. I have ten years of data that proves it 'just ain't so!' The solution is stunningly simple: to improve nursing homes, you have to improve nursing homes (not the inspection system) one professional at a time, one issue at a time, one facility at a time. At the end of the day, that is what it is going to take.

Why not invite a church to sponsor a program on quality elder care, and ask a local reporter to serve as your moderator? Include state inspectors and facility caregivers on a panel. Serve refreshments to create a cordial atmosphere. Begin to talk about improving care, one issue at a time.

TODAY: *Begin a dialogue.*

One last secret for the persecuted: the person taunting you is in much more pain than they could ever inflict on you.

To teach their children from being hurt by others, the Native Americans used legends. Little Raccoon, the mythical trickster, was always portrayed as a creature whose plots would backfire, putting him in a trap he set for someone else. Children learned "if one always sets out to do bad things to others, misfortune will fall back upon the evil perpetrator."

Little Raccoon decided he would stamp out sleeping Brother Fox's fire, so it would be out when he awoke. Instead, Brother Fox woke to Little Raccoon's screams that his tail caught on fire. In another story, one winter day Little Raccoon peeked into the beaver's lodge and had his nose frostbitten, which wouldn't have happened if he had kept his nose out of others' business.

While we may not see physical pain caused by traps, fires and frostbite, we can know that tormenters are nevertheless tormented. Once we recognize that their behavior is simply an expression of the inner turmoil they carry, these mean individuals lose all power and control in our lives. Great freedom awaits us when we see such incidents for what they actually are: public declarations of personal unhappiness.

Such awareness is like a vaccination: once it is present, you are immune to slings and arrows. Awakening to the true nature of such attacks, the kingdom of heaven is yours. See the pain of the persecutor and be compassionate.

TODAY: *Be compassionate.*

September: Rejoice, and be glad, for your reward in heaven is great

Through all the trials and tribulations of life, we are not supposed to forget to find joy. We are taught here to find reasons to rejoice, particularly after suffering. Rejoicing with others we also share pain, and are thus released from its grip. When shared, pain is diluted and joy multiplied.

Rarely does a moment present itself that is pain-free, scoured of all discomfort or disappointment. Waiting for the perfect day to play, when all of life's hardships have disappeared, we deny the world and ourselves much pleasure. Making time now to smile and applaud now, we beautify the environment. Like a bouquet of balloons, our lightness and sparkle brighten up the room.

How many times have we heard or said, "If I don't laugh, I'll cry?" Disease, terminal illness and death are part of the caregiver's day, sometimes threatening to sweep you into their wake. Far from being disrespectful, expressing joy is the ultimate tribute to life.

Joy is contagious. As a caregiver, you are a carrier, responsible for spreading infectious laughter and giggles, breathing new life into old and tired attitudes. In the midst of the gray sorrow, you affirm the uniqueness of individuals and celebrate life together. Here is the New Covenant, the way to secure world peace and international understanding.

Humor embraces all, and joy can erase enemy lines. In the middle of a difficult day, a silly song and dance lift the gloom. Where does such joy come from? "Out of the blue," we declare with thanks, the mysterious and loving heavenly blue.

Many of us live great distances from family. Grandchildren are often more than a day's drive away. Working with many grandparents, you see the pictures of their loved ones and hear stories of the latest growth spurt.

"Matthew can do all his multiplication tables!"

"My little Nathan scored the winning goal in his soccer game last week!"

Rather than curse the distance, why not hold a Grandchildren's Birthday Party? Each month, ask residents if they have any grandsons or granddaughters celebrating a birthday. Make a poster and declare a specific day Grandchildren's Birthday. Decorate with pictures of grandchildren and serve cake. With luck, you may be able to arrange a few surprise phone calls during the party, as well.

Rituals are the way we punctuate moments of our sacred time together. Fortunately, there are no rules about too many rituals or parties. Isn't it time for another?

TODAY: *Celebrate grandchildren's birthdays.*

Since 1894, Canada and the United States have officially celebrated Labor Day on the first Monday of September as the annual national tribute to the contributions workers have made to the strength, prosperity and well-being of our countries.

Samuel Gompers, founder and longtime president of the American Federation of Labor said:

> Labor Day differs in every essential way from the other holidays of the year in any country. All other holidays are in a more or less degree connected with conflicts and battles of man's prowess over man, of strife and discord for greed and power, of glories achieved by one nation over another. Labor Day...is devoted to no man, living or dead, to no sect, race, or nation.

Usually a quiet time for major news stories, Labor Day makes an excellent time for caregivers to appear in the media declaring dedication to their labor of love. Why not host an open house or cookout for the press and public to acquaint them with the joys of caregiving? Over hot dogs and cotton candy, tell the world why caring for others is such a blessing.

If such a big event is impractical, create a Shadow a Labor of Love Day, where youth are invited to spend time with you, learning what caregivers do. Provide prospective employees with first-hand evidence of the rewards they can expect when choosing a career in long-term care.

TODAY: *Celebrate your labor of love.*

St. Patrick's Residence in Naperville, Illinois, is one of the facilities owned and operated by the Carmelite Sisters of the Aged and Infirm. To honor the nursing assistants of St. Pat's, the staff planned a day of celebration around the theme, "CNAs are a Work of Heart."

The CNA Day program read:

> Jesus spent His short time on this earth doing many good deeds and performing miracles. While He preached to large crowds, He always gave compassionate care to individual needs, both physical and emotional. Jesus loved everyone. He showed his love in word and action.

> We believe that all of you, our CNAs, continue this healing ministry of Jesus. We are grateful for who you are and what you do.

Creating a special facility holiday for aides, St. Pat's provided all staff, residents and family members an opportunity to express joy and gratitude. Rallying around a theme, even shy family members were able to thank caregivers for making a great difference in their lives. By simply giving individuals a context for praising everyday acts of kindness, St. Pat's strengthened relationships and staff dedication.

TODAY: *Create CNA Day.*

One July, the staff at Rancho Mirage Health Care, in Rancho Mirage, CA, planned and hosted a Hawaiian Luau. Nursing assistant Julia Jones organized the outdoor celebration, dedicated to honoring Beverly care specialists and other area nursing assistants. Julia wrote:

> We invited CNAs from a 10-mile radius of our facility. We wanted to let them know how much the community appreciates what they do. While it wasn't easy, I was able to persuade a local television news crew to attend and film the event. Later that night, video of the luau was broadcast, showing viewers happy CNAs laughing, dancing and enjoying the festivities. I wonder if they had ever seen a CNA on the news that wasn't being charged with abuse, neglect or theft.

> Highlights of the luau were a whole roasted pig, complete with apple in his mouth, and a dunk tank. Our administrator and director of nursing services were the most popular dunk tank targets.

> Rancho Mirage has hosted other large, fun events to remind staff they are special and valued. An Employee Appreciation Awards ceremony patterned after Hollywood's Oscars was another success earlier this year.

> We encourage everyone to participate. Remember, there is no letter 'I' in the word 'team!'

TODAY: *Celebrate caregiving.*

The memory of a clever television commercial that aired in Belfast, Northern Ireland remains with me. A large, empty meeting room appears on-screen. An off-camera voice announces the anticipated arrival of representatives from all sides of the 700-year-old English/Irish dispute: "Delegates have been invited to gather today, to find common areas of agreement."

Suddenly, a toddler dressed only in a diaper crawls into the room. The baby is followed by another and then another, all giggling. Colorful balls roll across the floor. Nothing more is said. Viewers watch the joyful, spontaneous play of dozens of pre-schoolers, unaware of concepts such as "enemy" and "terrorist bombing."

Stripped of clothing's identifying characteristics, British and Irish babies were indistinguishable. Together, they reminded viewers how joyous life can be when peace prevails.

Joining a facility team, such as softball or bowling, is a great way to enjoy the company of fellow employees. Playing the game, it doesn't matter whether one has a college degree or has managed the laundry for ten years. Fun is the great leveler, the healer of foolish riffs.

TODAY: *Let fun heal.*

When you've loved being a nursing assistant for ten years, as has Sandra Allen of Lenexa, Kansas, you learn to enjoy a good laugh whenever it presents itself.

Sandra was caring for a retired Presbyterian minister, wheelchair-bound with badly arthritic knees. She recalls one morning: "I was getting him dressed, and had him stand so I could pull his trousers up. 'Oh my knees, I feel like an old man!' he said, causing us both to laugh."

One Saturday night, the preacher told staff "he was worried that he didn't have a Sunday sermon done yet." In recollecting this conversation, Sandra points out the fine line between laughing at and with a resident. And sometimes a smile is all that is needed.

"I took care of another resident who believed she was 16 years of age," Sandra wrote. "She had a colostomy bag she had named Genevieve. One morning, as I was getting her roommate dressed, I heard her in her bathroom, taking to the bag, giving it a civics lesson, and darned if she wasn't accurate. She was telling this appliance about the whole election process!"

TODAY: *Appreciate the moment.*

When it came to our childhoods, my mom was a saver. Besides baby teeth and hair, the attic was full of our schoolwork and art projects.

Cleaning out the attic when moving to a smaller home, my mom found a letter to the editor I wrote on Feb 2, 1962. I was just ten days from my 10th birthday, and already taking on the press:

> Dear Editor: I disagree with the article, 'No Early Spring.' My point is in the Friday paper, Feb. 2: 'Another 1.5 inches of snow were added to the almost two feet we accumulated in January. The new junk...

> Now my first point is the way you talk! You should set an example, and you should not talk about nature as 'junk.'

> My second point is, quote: 'that magical sign of the season dumped,' is that talking about our most important source of life (water) as being dumped is disrespectful. A newspaper should help people appreciate nature.

So there! Nearly 40 years later, I happen to think I did have a point! Our descriptive language does reveal what we feel. How do you talk about the individuals in your care? Do you choose respectful words that indicate appreciation and high regard? Do you recognize the privilege of your work, and speak accordingly?

TODAY: *Speak with appreciation.*

Prayer to the Creator of Life

Creator of the East Wind: we give you thanks. In you is each day's beginning, the spring of our lives, when we plant for our tomorrows. In you are our dreams for ourselves, our families and communities, and our sacred earth. In you are the gifts of early flowers. In you our children are born.

Creator of the South Wind: we give you thanks. In you are the summers of our lives, the long days of sunlight, and work where we build our homes and our gardens, where we teach our children what they must know to grow strong and secure. In you are gifts of warmth and giving, of growing into wholeness.

Creator of the West Wind: we give you thanks. In you are the days of harvest and the peace of coming home after life's journeys. In you are the lessons we have learned, put together with all the gifts of your people, the closing of days and the coming of night. In your are the glories of sunset and the songs of evening around the fire that is our heart and our life.

Creator of the North Wind: we give you thanks. In you are the days of winter, of closing down and coming into our homes, of snow that covers the earth with sleep. In your keeping are all those who have gone before us, who wait for us on the road ahead, who teach us through our dreams and visions. In you is our end, our peace, our eternity.

Creator of the earth, our home: we give you thanks. From your heart comes that which feeds your people, the gifts of plant and animals, our brothers and sisters, who walk with us in this journey toward you. By your abundant life, we are fed; by the living water that springs from deep within your being we drink.

Creator of the sky, the sun and moon of day and night, the stars that guide us in darkness: we give you thanks. Beneath the broad blanket of your presence we measure our days and our years. By the warmth of your sun we grow into our promise and vision; by the darkness at day's end we rest securely.

Creator of life, we give you thanks: you give us the gift of your people, our families both of birth and of choice, human love that secures the edges of life's blanket, human hands to hold and to teach us, human voices to join ours in prayer and song. In all life, both here and within your sacred eternal homeland, we are held in your hands.

This Abenaki Blessing was used by the native peoples who once populated southern Quebec and northern Vermont, where I live. Copy this blessing and read it standing, as a group, before a meal or staff meeting. As you read aloud, turn and face the direction mentioned.

TODAY: *Give thanks.*

Regardless of our age or circumstance, romance is a great cause for rejoicing. Marie is tickled by her widowed father's new love life. Terribly lonely after the death of his wife, Mr. Stone, age 83, made a lady friend at the swimming pool. The couple is now on a two-week vacation at Marie's. "My dad was always up, making the coffee at 6 AM," Marie says. "Now, I'm lucky if I see him by 11 AM!"

Hooray for love!

Three years after Linda McCartney's death, Beatle Paul could not imagine being with another woman. Until he met model Heather Mills, who had lost part of a leg in car accident. Presenting at a humanitarian awards program in Britain, the two met and fell in love. "He is so romantic," Heather said. "On Halloween he invited me to his house, where he had carved 20 pumpkins and had them all lit in a circle for me."

Finding a reason to love again following an incredibly painful loss is a courageous act for all parties. The lovers themselves risk all of the hazards brought on by comparisons. For their friends and family, the challenge is to resist passing judgment or condemning the new relationship. When relationships end, survivors cannot live on memories alone. New love is allowed, and is to be celebrated.

TODAY: *Celebrate new love.*

Curious children are a challenge, I know. I chaperoned my son's fifth grade class bus trip to Boston. After more than 12 hours of travel and adventure, it was dark and we were headed back to Vermont. Only the occasional shifting gears of the bus disturbed the night. We were all quiet, with lights out, except one little traveler: my son. "Mom, this is boring," he told me, complaining there was no one to play cards with but me.

Elliot and I weathered many such moments, and usually found fun ways to enjoy the time. I especially recommend the game Rename Me. Take someone's first and last name and scramble the letters to spell another name. Bethany Knight becomes Begin Thy Thank. Sitting next to my new friend Nicholas Dewey on a long bus ride in India, I christened him Wise Holy Dance or Clean Nose Daily!

During the dull, down times that can take over the day, introduce Rename Me to staff and residents. See what silly new identities you can invent. Discover ways to make one another laugh.

TODAY: *Play Rename Me.*

So how do you celebrate your professional anniversary? What's a professional anniversary? The day you became a caregiver—your first day on the job. Some caregivers have never left the original job or employer. Others have a varied trail of caring for different kinds of people in need.

In some ways, our professional anniversary is as important as our birthday. The day you answered your call and entered your profession, you began to grow in a new way. Every day you have cared for others, you have grown and evolved. You are not the same person you were starting out. You are not different; you are just more you, a deeper and more powerful you.

Make a list of everyone's anniversaries. You can decide as a group which date you want to honor, the day you began working where you are now, or going back to the first job.

In what clever and affordable ways can the facility celebrate your day? Create a ritual for rejoicing. Should associates be given their anniversary day off? Should they be allowed to wear casual clothes? Pick the facility menu? Have a cake? Wear a crown or costume? Have their picture on the front door of the building, inviting all visitors to share in the rejoicing? "On this date in 1979, a Caregiver Was Born!"

TODAY: *Celebrate anniversaries.*

"Mine has been an experience that has ripened into faith as strong as the hills; it has given me a hope that admits me into the room called Beautiful," wrote poet and songwriter Fanny Crosby. With 9,000 hymns to her credit, it is probable that no other human being has brought such musical help, solace, and peace to so many millions.

Born in 1820 in New York State, Frances Jane Crosby was scarcely more than six weeks old when she lost her sight; but the misfortune did not check the joyousness of her nature or restrain her activity. The gladness of heart, the resolute spirit, and the practical mind of the future woman are clearly foreshadowed in the following rhymes written when she was only eight years old:

Oh, what a happy soul I am,
Although I cannot see!
I am resolved that in this world
Contented I will be.
How many blessings I enjoy
That other people don't
To weep and sigh because I'm blind,
I cannot and I won't!

Fanny was already eleven before the first school for the blind was opened in the United States, and it was in the early years of the Institution in New York City that she received her education. After graduation, she went on to teach at the school and then to write hymns, so many she had to use a variety of pen names, to avoid hymnals all being written by one person!

Fanny wrote:

Where selfishness is happiness cannot be found. When I look down the avenue of these ninety years, I find that I have been interested in everything advanced for the welfare of mankind. I have made up my mind never to become a disagreeable old woman, and always to take cheer and sunshine with me.

On the evening of February 11, 1915, when she was almost ninety-five years of age, Fanny Crosby dictated a letter to cheer a bereaved friend, including a poem, which she recalled perfectly. She died before dawn.

TODAY: *Take cheer and sunshine with you.*

When we do something with enthusiasm, we should remember that the phrase literally means, "with God within."

Approaching the day with this level of pep and energy, we are truly alive, conveying a sense of shared divinity that pervades all creation. We are more than flesh and blood; we are co-creators of this beautiful day.

At a workshop in Nebraska, an enthusiastic personnel director thanked a group of nursing assistants for their years of service. She presented a goody bag to each CNA, full of clever reminders that proclaimed, "We rejoice in your service to others!"

Perhaps you would like to distribute some similar bags to coworkers?

Marker: To remind you to continue to make your mark as a leader by communicating what's important.

Mint: To remind you that you're worth a "mint" to all who know and love you!

Golden Thread: To remind you that your friendship and your kindness are a golden thread that ties our hearts together.

Lifesaver: To remind you that you are often a lifesaver to others, courageously standing up to negative statements that can steal an individual's sense of worth and damage a community.

Button: To remind you to "button your lip," and not waste your breath on frustrations or issues undeserving of your energy.

Eraser: To remind you that mistakes are unavoidable, and that you can always erase your embarrassment or disappointment by asking the forgiveness of yourself (or others) and moving on!

TODAY: *Enthusiastically rejoice.*

"We wrecked the house this weekend," Elliot told me with a chuckle. Paper-training his eight-week-old puppy, Sebastian, Elliot said the apartment was covered with newspapers, chewed pine cones, empty tea boxes and anything else Seb could sink his teeth into. "Just before Annie got home, we cleaned it all up!"

We rejoice when it is okay to make a mess. Healthcare facilities are held to rigorous standards, which sometimes makes the mess of living a bit tough.

Julia, my ward, and Jean, her roommate at the nursing home, share a big armoire with drawers at the bottom. I call it their Dress-Up Closet. No matter how many times staff sort, separate and fold their clothes, Julia and Jean can pull the whole thing apart in less than five minutes. Ideally matched, these two women love to try on clothes throughout the day, with no real attention to who owns what.

I am grateful to the staff of Union House for not making too big a deal out of keeping the Dress-Up Closet tidy. What matters to me is that Julia and Jean are happy and having fun, not that every sock is in its place.

I experienced the same sense of joyous freedom watching "the girls" do crafts one Sunday with Liz. Thanks to all caregivers who live and let live.

TODAY: *Rejoice in messes.*

Frances enjoys bingo, but to be honest, she enjoys winning most of all. An exceptionally alert resident at the nursing home, she plays multiple cards each game, doubling and tripling her chances to win. Frances suffers from a mental illness, making it impossible to live alone. Still, she enjoys a great deal of independence, and is often seen walking from the facility to the general store, just three doors down.

"Sister, have you tried those great hot dogs at Currier's?" she asked me one afternoon, beaming her joyous smile my way. "My are they good, you should really try one!"

"Did you just go down and buy a hot dog?" I asked.

"Oh yes, sister. Won fifty cents at bingo. My, was that hot dog good."

My mother has always enjoyed hot dogs at baseball games, talking about them in the same reverent terms as Frances. I am struck by the beauty and joy discovered in simple pleasures: a hot dog, an ice cream cone, a pinkish-orange sunset.

This is the day that the Lord hath made. Let us rejoice and be glad in it.

TODAY: *Enjoy simple pleasures.*

Working as a nursing assistant, I felt like a foreign exchange student at times, so unfamiliar with the ways and customs of this new world. Would I ever be able to take on such serious responsibility with such a light touch? With lives literally at stake, how did these extraordinary women and men manage to smile and stay at ease? I was afraid I would break people transferring them from the bed to the wheelchair.

Caregiving has its own rhythm and stride. Without question, knowing how to approach delicate and difficult situations takes experience and genius. Those who know Denise Anderson of Sebring, Florida have seen such talent in action. Named Nursing Assistant of the Year by the Florida Association of Nurse Assistants (FANA) in 2000, Denise has practiced her craft since 1975. In nominating Denise for the award, her supervisor, Becky McIntyre of the Heartland Home Health Agency, told this story:

> For the past several years, Denise has been one of the primary caregivers for one elderly client who lives alone, bed-bound, in his apartment. This gentleman's personality is at times very difficult. He is an ex-Marine and has a gruff manner.

> One evening, her supervisor called the client's home unexpectedly and heard Denise and the client giggling uncontrollably. When asked what was going on, Denise proceeded to tell her supervisor that they were blowing bubbles with containers of bubble solution.

> There are very few people who can get this client to smile, much less laugh and have fun. She provided a welcome break in his otherwise monotonous day. When this client was recently hospitalized, Denise went out of her way to make sure his favorite pillow and other personal belongs were taken to the hospital for him.

Gifted caregivers are treasured by all those who know them. Like Denise Anderson, they bring magic to the bedside.

TODAY: *Blow some bubbles.*

As mothers know, we simply can't keep an eye on our children every moment they are awake. Working in a healthcare residence, circumstances are similar, and comical surprises can result. While it seems caregivers have eyes in the back of their heads, unsupervised individuals still have a few adventures.

Visiting Julia at Union House one Sunday, I was getting ready to leave when I offered to take her to the bathroom. Yes, she would like my help. We've known one another for years, since before I became her guardian, and we're both comfortable with my playing the part of her aide.

Traveling with her walker and with a rather unsteady gate, Julia eventually made her way to the bathroom. "Would you like me to come in and help?" I asked, and she said "yes." Julia positioned herself over the toilet, and I proceeded to pull her pants down. "Why, Julia, you have no underwear on!" I exclaimed.

Appearing as surprised as I was, Julia let out a hoot. That got me laughing, and there we were, laughing like schoolgirls in the bathroom.

I know how hard the staff works to keep Julia dressed nicely. I also know she likes to change her outfits during the day, and guessed this outfit was one of her own choosing.

As I left, the staff promised to help Julia get fully dressed, and I said goodbye, a grin still on my face.

TODAY: *Laugh at surprises.*

All over the Western world, employers are searching for quality caregivers. How can there be such a shortage of people who care for people?

Of course there is no shortage. What we have is an increase in barriers to caregiving, making it tougher for women and men to consider such employment. The work has always been demanding both on physical and emotional levels; that's not new. And no one has ever made any real money as a direct care worker, either.

What's new is that the culture has turned on caregivers. The media regularly reports on poor care and lawsuits against caregivers are more common every day. When taken as a whole, these negative factors discourage individuals from joining the helping professions.

In Kansas, I met an amazingly cheerful nursing assistant who was wearing a colorful smock, covered with smiling teddy bears. "What an adorable top!" I said, "Where did you get it?"

"Oh, I made it. I make lots of them for staff at the home."

Listening to this woman's story gladdened my heart:

> I was working in a convenience store as a cashier, and the man who is the administrator of the nursing home kept telling me I should come and work for him. Every time he shopped, he would say I was such a happy person he wanted to have me on his staff. Finally, one day, I just gave in. And I love it!

I could immediately see what the administrator had seen, what everyone who meets the young aide notices: she is full of joy and good will. Despite all the barriers, the home was successful at bringing her on board. Look around for the smiling faces that greet you each day. Can any be persuaded to join your merry team of caregivers?

TODAY: *Look for smiling faces.*

Staff meetings are rarely cause for rejoicing. We're glad the paychecks are handed out, but that often backfires because employees sit like prisoners, waiting for the meeting to end. Checks have to be cashed and bills paid before the power or phone are cut off.

That's what made the Minnesota facility staff meeting so incredible. Called by Travis, the administrator, the meeting was for all the mentors working in the nursing department. Mentors are specially trained staff who oversee and support new nurses and aides, making sure they successfully perform their duties.

"Get on the bus, we're going to a comedy club," Travis told his bewildered crew. A comedy club?

"Yes, we all need a good laugh and a change of scenery," the young administrator explained. The light-hearted outing was the best of medicine. Friendships were forged that day, and the team was solidified. Objectively speaking, isn't that what a good staff meeting should accomplish?

Written announcements of policy changes can be distributed and discussed as needed. But no paperwork can be circulated to create relationships or bonds. Getting to know one another happens in a relaxed, fun setting.

How can you liven up your staff meetings? Can you pull a few other associates together and perform a skit which communicates an important policy or procedure? Can the kitchen provide just-out-of-the-oven cookies? Can the day care children lead you in the pledge of allegiance? Find ways to bring a smile and create moments for rejoicing, even at the most boring of staff meetings.

TODAY: *Liven up staff meetings.*

For more than a week, pink posters had been hanging throughout the facility, announcing the upcoming visit of a gifted ballet dancer. "We are blessed to have Madame Candy Niveb with us Wednesday morning, to perform a series of impromptu dances."

"Who is Madame Candy Niveb?" staff and residents asked. The administrator said he wondered about whether the ballerina could visit while she was in the area. "I don't know anything about ballet, but I figured we all could use a lift this time of year."

Mr. Bevin was right about the need for a mood elevator. A bad bout of the flu had run through the building the last few weeks. Three residents had died. Some staff members were still out sick. Special entertainment would certainly help take everyone's minds off the tough stuff.

Wednesday after breakfast, Mr. Bevin announced over the intercom that Madame Candy Niveb was headed for the lobby. "Let's all give her a big Glen Lake Welcome!"

Staff and residents filled the dining hall. "I'm telling you, this is no big deal," said one female resident. "One dancer can't do that much alone."

But this one sure did. Candy Niveb was none other than 240-pound administrator Ed Bevin (Niveb spelled backwards) in a pink net tutu and blond wig. With a basket of candy, he flitted around the room, liberally sharing his chocolate kisses. The crowd loved it!

TODAY: *Lift spirits.*

Tickling my son when he was a little boy was so much fun! I loved his cascading giggles; just hearing him would make me laugh.

Once in a while, perhaps when all the planets are perfectly aligned, we hear or see something funny and our laughter explodes. The more we try to stop laughing, the funnier the incident becomes. Whatever worries or stresses we might have been carrying are washed away in the silliness.

"Tom had told us to have our summer vacation requests in by Friday, or he could not guarantee we would get our first choice of dates," Kitty recalled. A small facility, it was always a bit tricky scheduling staff time off.

"That Friday about 3 PM, Sue Anne came running down the hall toward Tom," Kitty recalled.

"I've got my vacation request form right here. It's due today, right?" Sue Anne said, handing the paperwork to the administrator.

"Yes, that's right, Sue Anne. Let's see," Tom scanned the form, "What dates are you requesting? You haven't written in any actual dates you want off."

"Well," Sue Anne answered, "I don't know what I want off yet, but you said we had to get our requests in today, if we wanted to get our first choice."

Overhearing this nonsensical conversation from her office, Kitty began to chuckle, and she couldn't stop. "The more I thought about it, the harder I laughed," she said, recalling the confused look on Tom's face.

TODAY: *Get the giggles.*

Years ago, a young man could always find a job pumping gas. But the invention of self-serve gas stations changed all that. Even more years ago, cowboys roamed the range, herding cattle across the great plains of the West. History tells us that the invention of barbed wire fencing put 8 out of every 10 cowboys out of work.

Technology is forever altering our world, with new ways to be more efficient and less dependent on people. Think of all the telephone operators who used to place our long-distance telephone calls. Like gas pump jockeys and cowboys, those jobs are gone with the wind.

The good news is that if you're a caregiver, you always will be needed. You will never be without work. From the Civil War for almost one hundred years, orphanages could be found throughout the United States. Caregivers were needed in these institutions to care for children orphaned by war, disease and abandonment. In the 1960s, smaller group homes became a more popular model for providing childcare, and the orphanages gradually closed.

Did that leave caregivers without work? No! Nor did the closing of the great mental hospitals of this nation. Because no matter the latest model for providing care, caregivers are still needed.

What a comfort! You will never be considered obsolete, a thing of the past, a relic of earlier days! Even if you move to another part of the country, your skills as a caregiver are in demand. On those days you need a reason to rejoice, remember your job security. Technology may replace a lot of people and positions, but you are here to stay.

TODAY: *Celebrate job security.*

During the admission process in a nursing home or assisted living facility, lots of issues are covered. For the family members helping their loved ones make this big move, the strain is obvious.

The stress that built up to the day is usually tremendous, as leaving home is not a simple decision, particularly for an older person. Helping parents or a spouse make the transition from the familiar to the unknown is demanding. Sometimes it seems nothing can be done or said to reduce the shock.

Working with families as they enter this new world, gifted caregivers can ease the moment with little or no fanfare. After all, the move isn't just from one building to another; it includes the bonus of now being served by compassionate caregivers.

As caregivers, welcoming a new resident in not a traumatic event full of dread and resistance. Your life's work is about reaching out and making peace. Rather than focusing on what is lost in the move, you can help the family recognize what they are about to gain—an expansion of their family. Yesterday there were fewer people who cared about their loved one than there are today. Today, you and your colleagues have been added to the list. And unlike family members, you consciously chose this line of work: this is your vocation. (You even enjoy the challenge of getting a grouchy resident to grin!)

New residents usually struggle with a move into a health-care facility, while their families often experience a great sense of relief. As the professional caregiver in the equation, it is your responsibility to remind all parties of the need to rejoice. A good, loving home has been found. You are here to care. Everything will be all right. Suggest that for the next visit they bring some photo albums so you can get a feel for the family you are joining. You need to get to know everyone who shares a love for your new resident.

TODAY: *Remind families to rejoice.*

"Kooky" is a word that can be used for some of the down-right odd things that happen when two or more people gather. Caregivers are well aware of the streaks of strangeness that run through a facility. With so many people under one roof, of course something unusual will happen.

At Countryside Place in Mishawaka, Indiana, home of the world's finest caregivers, they like to talk about Mary, the resident who gives staff nicknames. No one can explain for sure how Mary's titles are cooked up or bestowed; it just happens.

Sue, the RN who handles all of the paperwork for the resident assessments, tells of the pet name she was assigned:

"I've just always been Sue Charise. I don't know why—that's just what she's called me. Now everybody calls me that. I think a lot of people believe Charise is actually my last name."

When Sue goes home at the end of the day, Mary, the Naming Fairy sings out, "Sue Charise has left the building!" Everyone understands.

"Once I received a phone call, and Ann paged me as 'Sue Charise,'" Sue laughs. And why not? Part of the unique color and flavor of Countryside Place is the fun, loving energy that flows through the conversations and interactions of the day. Wise caregivers, these folks have learned to never turn down a chance to smile.

TODAY: *Enjoy the unusual.*

Big groups of nursing homes are like a country of many states. Yes, California and Florida are both members of the republic, but they seem so far away, with so little reason to communicate.

For the staff in the company's headquarters, this feeling of disconnection can be even more intense. Clerks in the corporate office spend eight hours a day organizing paperwork and data, a lifetime away from the heart of the business, caring for people in need.

To be content, human beings need to feel useful, to have meaning in their lives. Knowing one has correctly alphabetized a list of accounts may not be enough to generate job satisfaction. To heighten the home office staff's awareness of its indirect contribution to the well-being of elderly residents, Beverly Healthcare began a pen pal program.

The brainchild of an associate in the Fort Smith, Arkansas headquarters, the voluntary program links caregivers in the field with corporate office workers. Receiving a letter from a nursing assistant about her day, her pen pal feels closer to the company's mission and vision. A greater sense of team and purpose is created, uniting groups who once were estranged.

Recognizing we belong to something larger than ourselves is exhilarating. No longer do we regard our own efforts as isolated and of little value. With an awareness of where we fit into the larger picture, we have reason for pride and joy. Whatever your job working for a healthcare provider, rejoice knowing you help others.

TODAY: *Recognize you belong.*

"I always plan the parties, and I'm getting sick of it!"

Sometimes the same people are asked to plan all of the social events, and usually because they are good at the assignment. Still, resenting involvement in what should be a joyous occasion is not healthy.

Equally dangerous is the habit of keeping track of who did what for whom, tit-for-tat bookkeeping: "I'm not giving her a birthday card until she gives one to me!"

Whenever we begin to feel this biting sense of being wronged over what should be a happy situation, it's time to step back and reflect. Get back to the basics, and remember why a celebration is desired in the first place. What milestone or achievement is being honored? How much does it mean to the celebrant?

Hosting a party or giving a gift are not acts to be practiced out of obligation. If you don't feel right about getting involved in the special time, don't get involved. Let someone else step forward to lead the rejoicing. Faking a laugh is bad enough, but faking a party is unacceptable.

TODAY: *Rejoice honestly.*

Life certainly is what we make it. Ask anyone who has dieted. Delicious fresh fruit and low-fat cheeses are a lot more interesting than drinking the same can of chocolate something every noon hour.

I remember how, as a single mom, it was so hard to get my son to sit for more than seven minutes for supper. Putting a sheet on the living room floor and announcing a picnic always bought me at least three more minutes!

Using a little creativity we can add zing to routines, shining up the dullness of a day. Some physical therapists are sheer geniuses at making fun out of boring and repetitious exercises.

"Parade 11 AM" was printed on the activities calendar. Those who weren't in the parade were stationed in the facility hallways, along the route, waving colored cloth pennants they had made the week before. Out of the physical therapy room came the parade master, dressed as Uncle Sam and pushing his wheelchair, decorated as a float. In the wheelchair a boom box broadcast marching music. The parade was in full swing!

With walkers, canes or an aide at their side, the physical therapy patients moved through the big building with joy. Spectators received them with equal glee. What a grand way to make sure rehabilitation clients walked their 50 or 100 feet! And what a reminder to us all to make the absolute most out of all we have.

TODAY: *Organize a parade.*

Shoes make great conversation pieces. My husband likes to talk about not owning a pair of shoes until he started school at age six. He still loves to walk barefoot in the cool grass on a summer morning.

Helping residents dress in the morning is a perfect time to talk about their first pair of shoes. Were they hand-me-downs? Did someone teach them how to tie a bow in the laces? Did they have to wear them until they wore out? Did they buy shoes for their babies? Knit booties? Have baby shoes bronzed?

In my family, we received a new pair of shoes at the beginning of the school year. I kept mine in the shoebox in my closet, inhaling the smell of new leather and feeling a tingle of excitement about school starting soon. I remember my first September living on my own, wondering if I should go and buy a pair of shoes or not.

Whatever clothing item or piece of jewelry you decide to focus on, spend time talking to your residents about their memories. Is that their wedding ring? Can they tell you about it? Was it a family heirloom or purchased new, just for them? Can they remember an especially happy and beautiful fall day? Discover facts about one another; find reasons to recall moments of joy.

TODAY: *Reminisce and rejoice.*

On the blackboard outside the activities room, the note read "Rabbi In Room. Don't Open Door."

New to the facility, the visitor was intrigued. I wonder what the rabbi is doing here, she thought. How wonderful that he visits.

"I'm here to drop off some donations for the rummage sale," the visitor told the receptionist. "My daughter said I could leave them in the activities room, but I can't open the door."

The receptionist looked puzzled. "It's not locked, is it?"

"No. The sign says the rabbi is in there and not to open the door."

"The rabbi? Um, just a moment."

The activities director was paged and questioned. Gales of laughter followed.

"Ma'am, there's a rabbit in the room and they don't want it to escape. Somebody must have smeared that sign!"

The rabbi tale made its way through the building, with the same effect on all listeners. What is more healing that a good joke?

Human beings love to hear laughter. Working for years at a facility, you are known by your laugh. Even without seeing you, coworkers and residents hear your laugh and know you are around. Make time for jokes and fun. Life is never too busy for a laugh.

TODAY: *Pass a laugh.*

We live in a time when half of all marriages end in divorce. Companies no longer reward employees after 20 or 30 years with a watch, but with a pink slip for lay-off.

Are the days of lifelong commitments gone? Not totally.

What do swans, beavers, Canadian geese, moose and wolves have in common? They mate for life. No matter how the modern world has changed around them, these creatures remain true to their species.

Within your circle at work, there are people who have remained true to their spouses and work. Many of your residents have celebrated 50 years of marriage, or more. Many of your coworkers have worked at the facility since they left high school. Other employees come and go, but these individuals are your anchors, keeping standards and history from drifting away.

Is it time to create and celebrate a new holiday, Old-Timer's Day? Get the activities department involved, and ask them about making some fancy ribbons to award as prizes. Decorate with a swan or a moose! Make up some categories for winners, such as "longest-serving aide on A-wing," or "nurse with the most experience on the night shift."

How about acknowledging some incredible achievements among the residents? Perhaps a ribbon for best citizen— someone who has voted in every election since they were of age? If you are creative enough, every person in the building will end up with a ribbon recognizing their commitment to something of value.

With so many winners and such commitment, what can you do but call the newspapers and tell them you've got a great story to tell? Maybe let the Guinness Records people know, too, that yours is a home where people don't give up!

TODAY: *Honor commitment.*

October: You are the salt of the earth.

"Salt is born of the purest of parents: the sun and the sea."
—Pythagoras

Without salt, life as we know it would not exist. Salt gives life, reminding us that all comes from the sea. The same percentage of salt-to-water exists in the ocean, in blood, in sweat, in tears and in urine. Without salt, blood won't circulate, food won't digest and hearts won't beat.

Found on land and in the sea, salt is the only rock consumed by man. Worth its weight in gold, salt has played a vital role in nearly every civilization since the beginning of time.

Your salty ministry is rooted in these mysterious and life-giving properties. You are essential to the spinning of the earth; your rock-solid loving presence can't be duplicated by a machine. You are real, a straight shooter, a truth teller, a life affirmer. You bring zest and flavor to all encounters.

Serving others in the noble vocation of caregiving, you seek to preserve and improve. Just as salt preserves food from decay and corruption, you stabilize environments. In your salty presence, there is less upheaval and cutting of corners, for you are a deterrent. You don't correct or reform, you simply lead by example.

Salt and caregiving run through our history and veins, linking the ages. They are essential to the life of plants and animals, to man's spiritual and material worlds.

Essential to the spiritual

Buddhists believe salt repels evil spirits.

Shinto practitioners use salt to purify, tossing a handful into a room before gatherings.

Pueblo Indians worshiped the Salt Mother.

Covenants in the Old and New Testaments were sealed with salt, the origin of the word salvation.

In Slavic countries, salt is given to a bride and groom to symbolize health and happiness.

In 1933, the thirteenth Dalai Lama was buried sitting on a bed of salt.

Essential to the material

Ancient Greeks exchanged slaves for salt—hence the phrase "not worth his salt."

Romans paid soldiers with salt rations known as "salarium argentum," the forerunner of the English word "salary."

Many governments, such as the early Chinese, knew salt was vital, so they made salt taxes a major revenue source.

Ancient Ethiopians used salt disks as a form of currency.

To sell salt, Arab traders carved the earliest trading routes around the world.

> But if the salt has become tasteless, how will it be made salty again? It is good for nothing anymore, except to be thrown out and trampled under foot by men.

As a stable compound, salt doesn't undergo chemical changes. Instead it mixes with or is diluted by other materials, becoming "good for nothing." Man cannot live without salt or caregivers. Many have lost their lives in war and peace due to a lack of salt. Without the small amount of salt needed by each human body, death occurs.

If you cease your salty ministry, and stop being yourself, what happens? What happens if you forget to take care of yourself? You can no longer take care of others. Life spoils; all becomes tasteless. You are the salt of the earth.

The late film star and comedienne Mae West said of herself, "I'm no model lady. A model's just an imitation of the real thing."

Patients can tell you what a pleasure it is to be cared for by the real thing—a caregiver who is a whole person. Unafraid of serving the whole patient, real caregivers handle circumstances with grace and style.

When Audrey was a young woman, her mother-in-law said it was time to get a job. "I'm going to take you to the Little Sisters," she told Audrey. "You can work for them."

"We drove up to the nursing home. I looked at her and said, 'What's this? I thought you were taking me to a dress shop!'" Audrey recalled with a laugh. "I had never heard of the Little Sisters of the Poor."

Thirty-five years later, Audrey is one of the veteran nursing assistants at the huge long-term care facility outside of Cleveland. Whenever she mentions retirement, the folks living on her floor say, "You can't leave until I die!"

Clearly beloved by all who know her, Audrey is a natural caregiver who returns all the love she receives. Her practice looks effortless; residents are bathed and dressed to a beat only Audrey can hear. In her care, men and women experience security they haven't enjoyed since childhood.

Dress sales would have been far too limiting for Audrey. She clearly needed to connect with others on a heart-to-heart level, grounded in the salt of the earth.

TODAY: *Be the real thing.*

Doing what's right isn't complicated, but it can be hard.

Marguerite loved her work as a nursing assistant. A confident and conscientious worker, she exuded grandmotherly warmth. Relationships were her specialty, which is why the situation with Denise had gotten unbearable: "We work together; she's the nurse on my shift. I can't remember why now, but we haven't talked to each other in a long time."

Recognizing what their stubborn stalemate was doing to the atmosphere, Marguerite made a decision. Who was at fault was no longer important, and digging up the past wasn't going to help. Resident care was obviously suffering with no communication between the two. The time had come to resume a working relationship with Denise.

Walking into work the next morning, Marguerite found Denise. "Hello, Denise."

"Hello."

The next day, Marguerite repeated her greeting and received the same response from Denise.

On day three, to Marguerite's "hello," Denise offered, "Hello, Marguerite."

On day four, before Marguerite could utter a word, Denise beat her to it. "Hello, Marguerite!"

Reflecting on this thaw, Marguerite said she didn't think she and Denise would ever be close friends. "But we are cordial to one another," she said, "and we're going to be able to talk about our patients' needs. That's what I feel good about."

Do you need to thaw some ice? Would resident care improve?

TODAY: *Thaw relations.*

Don't quit.
When things go wrong, as they sometimes will,
When the road you're trudging seems all uphill,
When the funds are low and the debts are high,
And you want to smile, but you have to sigh,
When care is pressing you down a bit,
Rest if you must, but don't you quit.
Life is queer with its twists and turns,
As every one of us sometimes learns,
And many a failure turns about,
When he might have won had he stuck it out.
Don't give up though the pace seems slow—
You may succeed with another blow.
Success is failure turned inside out—
The silver tint of the clouds of doubt.
And you never can tell how close you are.
It may be near when it seems so far.
So stick to the fight when you're hardest hit—
It's when things seem worst that you must not quit.

—Anonymous

TODAY: *Stay salty.*

We women are gloriously unique individuals, and vive la difference. However, it seems that on one subject virtually all women seem to agree: we love Judge Judy!

Judge Judith Sheindlin is the star of a televised courtroom show, "where the cases and people are real." We admire her strong qualities: how she says what is on her mind and exercises such common sense. Disputes between husbands and wives, as well as ex-girlfriends and ex-boyfriends, are daily fare in her court. Listening to the particulars of yet another domestic drama, Judge Judy quickly points out flawed thinking and ignorant behavior in her own no-nonsense style.

"Does it say 'idiot' across my forehead?" she asks a nervous witness who has given her a less-than-satisfactory answer. From our living room chairs, women of all ages and sizes are cheering the judge for not letting the defendant get away with anything. "Mr. Jones, are you stupid?" she asks.

Can you imagine blurting that question at someone, with no thought of the consequences? Judge Judy's courtroom environment allows her to be bold and impatient. After all, she is the judge and she holds the power.

Since my own pet peeve is men not replacing the toilet paper when it runs out, I especially love her joke: How many men does it take to change a roll of toilet paper? Answer: No one knows; it's never been done.

Back at the ranch, living in the real world, we cannot mimic Judge Judy's pronouncements and survive the consequences. People don't talk to one another the way Judge Judy talks to the litigants. Still, we can learn a lot from her ability to listen and assess a situation. Not being judges, we must deliver our message in a different style, yet still with strength and confidence. Your goal is not to entertain or get the last word, but to communicate accurately and respectfully.

TODAY: *Be strong and confident.*

Do you begin a diet every Monday and end it by Wednesday? Yo-yo dieting, in which weight is gained and lost and gained again constantly, is worse than not dieting at all. Researchers analyzed over 3,000 health records of the famous Framingham Heart Study and found those with fluctuating weights had a 75 percent greater risk of dying from heart disease than those whose weights remained stable.

In another piece of amazing research, rats were starved to 80 percent of their normal weight. When allowed to eat freely, they ate slightly less than their free-feeding littermates and yet gained weight 18 times as quickly!

Quality caregivers all too often put themselves last. Well-earned breaks are forsaken in favor of fixing a favorite resident's hair or making sure Mr. James successfully dials his son on the phone. While such sacrifices are above reproach, over time they can cause harm. Caregivers need to adopt the same level of compassion and commitment to themselves as they carry for others. Hydration, a balanced diet, exercise and rest are important for resident and caregiver alike.

Standing in the break room and inhaling a cupcake from the snack machine or gulping down a soda with chips will not fuel your machine. Later in the day, your body will send this message by delivering a headache or stomachache.

Acknowledging one's worthiness is a giant step in the life of a caregiver. Far from being a selfish act, the practice of disciplined self-care further honors the profession. Being attentive to your needs communicates to the patient that they deserve to receive the best, from the best.

TODAY: *Care for yourself.*

"I like to wear costumes all different times of year, not just Halloween," Donna laughed. A petite, energetic young woman, she said her favorite disguise for work was an elf outfit. No one at the workshop seemed surprised; Donna looked like an elf!

Getting to know each other's unique nature and interests is one of the great pleasures of caregiving. How many other workplaces would welcome Donna the Elf without hesitation? What other lunch hours could feature Jerry the dietary aide singing songs he wrote for the guitar?

Dealing daily with genuine issues of life, caregivers become comfortable with what is real. When a person in your care says, "I have to tell someone this secret, and I've decided to tell you," you accept the responsibility and honor without blinking.

Among the beautiful gifts of a caregiving career is the opportunity to fully be oneself and to be with others who are also being themselves. Without pretense or phoniness, you carry on as all compassionate souls have done through the ages. Yours is most privileged and sacred position: serving others as they complete their last great chapter of life.

TODAY: *Be yourself.*

The first time we meet another person, we have their attention as we never will again. Genevieve Gipson, founder and executive director of the National Network of Career Nursing Assistants, tells her members to have their introductory talk ready.

What do we want people to know about us? What message do we want to deliver during these precious, once-in-a relationship minutes? When you begin to recognize the power of initial conversations and all that is at stake, what you say becomes very important.

"Hello, I'm Rosie. I'm just a nurses' aide." Pretty weak.

"Hello, I'm Rosie and my life work is about caring for others. I've been a professional nursing assistant for six years." Now you've got their attention.

In our nervousness, we tend to waste our first words, throwing them away by whining about the weather or sharing some other complaint. Looking for a quick bond, we tend to put each other at ease with negative energy and finding a mutual enemy. But these lightweight connections create a false security, like an imitation Rolex watch. To begin a true friendship with someone, we need to give voice to meaning. Real ease comes when we are in the presence of beauty and truth, meeting the one and only you, not hearing some cheap knockoff conversation.

Watch your opening words. Go to the highest possible level to find common ground. Practice your introductory talk and have it ready.

TODAY: *Make your words count.*

To me, CNAs have one of the most physically draining jobs in the world. And yet, I've witnessed so many little acts of kindness and caring. Everything from making sure a particular resident has the special sundry she needs to buying treats with your own money. You dress residents in their nicest outfits, including jewelry for the holidays, birthdays and other special events.

Being blessed to have my parents here I have had the pleasure to observe numerous acts of human compassion and kindness from the CNAs: Caring Nurturing Angels. They are the Guardian Angels and the backbone of care with the sharp eyes and ears for safety—the strong arms and backs for the hard, backbreaking work. Plus they take time to listen and offer companionship and friendship.

CNAs are the heroes on the frontline of invaluable duty. They are doing the Lord's work and will be eternally rewarded. The heart and soul of a CNA is knowing that the resident one day could be their parents or loved ones, or themselves. I'm sure at the end of time, there will be a special place in heaven for CNAs. For truly, 'whatever you did for one of these, you did unto me.'

Thanks to Sister Del Ray of St. Patrick's Residence in Naperville, Illinois, for passing along these golden words of gratitude from family members of nursing home residents.

Rest assured that these appreciative families speak for the families of your residents as well. You are part of an age-old, sacred order of beings who have made the incredibly difficult and easy decision to devote their lives to others. For your gracious sacrifice, families hold you in their debt and cry out THANKS!

TODAY: *Hear family gratitude.*

In his world-famous depiction of the Last Supper, Leonardo da Vinci painted an overturned bowl of salt on the table in front of Judas. As we know, after this final meal with Jesus, Judas went on to betray him, to become salt without taste.

Betrayal is painful. Having entrusted someone with a secret, a fear or even our lives, we need to believe our message will be honored. Learning otherwise, we become confused, wondering how to behave, what to say.

When betrayal occurs, the circumstances are usually beyond our control. Rather than dwelling on the painful incident, the mature caregiver uses the event to look at his or her own life. Ask yourself: where is there falseness in my life? Where have I permitted hypocrisy?

My husband pointed out to me that I had answered a woman on the phone by telling her what she wanted to hear, rather than what I actually believed. "You smoothed that over, but you really didn't explain your differences," he said. "Did you really mean what you said?"

I got mad at him for his accusation, but it didn't take me long to recognize he was right. Playing up to another person by delivering a less-than-honest answer doesn't serve anyone. By not answering my friend with the truth, I betrayed her trust and my own conscience. I spilled the salt, failing to live up to my own standards of friendship and honesty.

Life is hard enough to accept and negotiate without further scrambling the day with inaccurate or twisted statements. Let's work together to keep the planet spinning in some regular orbit we can all count on. Let's loyally serve one another and the truth.

TODAY: *Be loyal to the truth.*

The morning started off a little frustrating for me as I put on my work shoes with a hole in the bottom of them. I just had discovered I needed (wanted) both cat food and smokes and could only afford one of them (the cat food won out—at least for today), wishing I earned more money on my way to work, wondering if it's really worth it.

YES! YES! YES! That answer came to me when I went in to wake up O'Dell. She led a vital life as a Hollywood extra in many musicals, had a wonderful life back then —and often wonders out loud what happened to it. She has three grown sons who never come to see her and she is well aware that one of them only lives two blocks away.

I've always had so much fun 'playing' with O'Dell as she plays with me, too. Anyway, as I was wondering about my job's worth while waking her up she said to me: "Did you know that when you walk into my room, or whenever I first see you every day, that that's when I start to live. I see your happy face, that twinkle in your eye and your happiness and sunshine just jumps right into my soul—I'm so happy that the good Lord saw fit to make you part of my life—you make me feel alive. I love you so very, very much."

Ah, yes, once again the fringe benefits make my modest wages worth it. Once again, I think I know why I'm here.

—Toni Tollestrup, CNA,
Lodi, California

TODAY: *Know why you're here.*

"I'm too lazy to brush my teeth tonight," I told my room-mate, Betty Blouin, as I headed for bed. We were on a peace pilgrimage and sharing a room.

"You are not too lazy, Bethany," Betty replied, "don't talk about yourself that way."

Betty was right. Negative self-talk had leaked into my thinking, and I wasn't being nice to myself. Once Betty flagged this bad habit, I began to notice other times and ways I did not speak about myself with kindness.

Teachers of meditation refer to thoughts flying through the mind as a monkey jumping from tree to tree, aimlessly in motion. When we slow down our thoughts to meditate, we create a stillness that leads to a deeper level of quiet. Without the constant chatter of the mind, we experience peace that passes all understanding.

Becoming more conscious of the mind's background noise can be both healing and freeing. For me, coming from a family where staying busy and being productive is prized behavior, my talk about being lazy reflects years of training. Without even cuing up the old music, these oldies but goldies play in my head all day long!

I thanked Betty for awakening me to my poor self-treatment, and reminded myself I was not lazy, just very tired. I certainly didn't need more self-criticism for being critical! Being gentle and loving with myself is not second nature yet, but I know I deserve positive self-talk. Sometimes I imagine I'm with little girl Bethany and I ask, "What do you need to hear today?"

TODAY: *Practice positive self-talk.*

When my friend and neighbor Bethany Dunbar, editor of Vermont's largest weekly paper, the *Barton Chronicle*, was 19, she worked for two months as the laundry girl in a local nursing home. Here's an excerpt from a poem she wrote at that time:

The Laundry Girl

Once
When Hazel was sitting in the hall,
She looked at me with those sharp
Little black eyes
And she grabbed my wrist tight.
"Is that you, Jesus?"
I said, no I'm just
the laundry girl.
Sometimes they get her
To saying the Lord's Prayer
So fast she
Sounds like an auctioneer.
And sometimes she
Just says,
"A one an' a two
an' a three an' a four
an' a five an' a six
an' a seven an' a eight."
She keeps going till
she loses her place.

Writing a poem helped young Bethany Dunbar deal with the sense of craziness she experienced in the nursing home. New employees, particularly ones who haven't seen a lot of life, can be overwhelmed and even frightened by what they see and hear their first month on the job. As a seasoned veteran, you can make time to help them absorb the experiences and work through their reactions. Casually check in with the greenhorns. Listen and laugh with them. Help them understand the many faces of aging.

TODAY: *Make sense of craziness.*

Our fascination with wizards and magicians is ancient. Transforming lead into gold and finding the secret of eternal life has fixated generations.

Medieval alchemists also tried to fabricate "prima materia" or "first matter." Possessing great patience and daring, the alchemist was a mix of scientist and magician. His goal was to duplicate the original raw material of life, from which he could make the philosopher's stone. Equipped with this stone, the alchemist could create anything.

Working with mercury and sulphur, the distilling process was completed by the addition of a third agent—salt: "Adding salt to the raw material makes the transformation complete. From the salt grain grows the philosopher's stone."

How wonderfully poetic to consider a grain of salt the seed from which all new life springs! Witnessing the transformation that occurs between a depressed, newly admitted resident and devoted caregiver makes believing in miracles easy.

Therese, an aide and my friend, routinely tells me of morose men and women who have just moved into the facility. "They don't want us to talk with them or touch them. They don't want to answer any questions; they just want to be left alone or they get mad."

Little by little, with her gentle, magical ways, Therese respectfully enters into their lives. From the tiniest little particle of common humanity, Therese and other caregivers of her caliber build a relationship. Before long, I receive another phone call: "Remember that little French man who wouldn't come out of his room?" she asks me.

"Today, we spoke French, and he asked about the dog that comes to visit."

Transformation! What creative genius lies in the hearts of caregivers?

TODAY: *Transform.*

Author and teacher Hanna Kroeger wrote "Ten Commandments for Good Health" that go beyond the physical and into the unseen world. "Observe them and enjoy perfect health," she promises!

1. Accept criticism as the other person's problem, not yours.

2. Appreciate yourself and reaffirm your self-worth whenever necessary.

3. See the good points in circumstances. See even problems as happening for the best.

4. Rather than looking backward with sorrow, look forward with joyous expectation.

5. Rather than fretting about what you do not have, appreciate what you have.

6. Learn from mistakes so that you can convert them into triumphs.

7. Insulate yourself from distasteful surroundings through wholesome detachment.

8. Let go of what you no longer need, and make the most of what you now attract.

9. Grow in courage and self-mastery from every circumstance.

10. Be aware of the larger consciousness of which you are a part.

Would you add or subtract anything? Go ahead and draw up your own commandments for good caregiver health. Invite coworkers and residents to join you. Hang up everyone's recommendations. Wallpaper the halls with recipes for healthy living!

TODAY: *Create healthy commandments.*

"If they do sell this building, what will happen to us? Will we keep our jobs with the new owner?" Amanda had been an aide for less than a year, she was just getting into the swing of things and comfortable with the job. Partnered with Trudy, one of the longest-serving CNAs on the schedule, Amanda whispered her worries.

"My father-in-law heard they were selling this place. I need this job, Trudy!"

In her fifties, Trudy had been through two building sales, four changes in administrators, her divorce and her daughter's divorce. "Amanda, honey, let me tell you something about change. It happens. And you live through it. Things always have a way of working out, even if you can't see it at the beginning. Just keep coming to work and doing the good job you do."

Able to look at this new situation through the wise eyes of experience, Trudy knows worrying about "what ifs" is pretty pointless. Not that she isn't still open to surprises—they are out there. But taking life one day at a time, she can handle surprises much more easily.

Projecting ahead and conjuring up horrible scenarios with awful outcomes isn't good for caregiver or patient health. Stay focused on what you know, which is providing excellent care, regardless of conditions or circumstances.

TODAY: *Focus on today.*

Teaching the valuable lessons of the Old Testament, Jewish rabbis insist that rest, specifically on the seventh day or the Sabbath, is essential for three reasons:

1. Rest equalizes everyone. On this one day, we are all the same, rich and poor alike. Neither striving nor struggling, we are aware of the same quiet and stillness, present in the same moment with our God.

2. Rest gives us time to evaluate our work. By stopping all activity, we can pause and reflect on what has been happening. Why do you feel tense or uptight? Why sad? Are you taking good care of yourself? Even God didn't work on the seventh day, preferring to evaluate his own performance. Surely you deserve a time-out and an opportunity to survey the week.

3. Rest provides time to contemplate the meaning of life. Is life limited to waking, eating, working, sleeping and starting over again? Or is there something greater and more beautiful going on, a preciousness that permeates each minute? If we take the Sabbath literally, and use Sunday to reflect, in 70 years we will have experienced 3,640 days of life review, or 10 years of Sabbath. Like taking a moment to read the map, a Sabbath day allows you to study your path and the journey you are on. Do you need to alter your direction? Speed? Destination?

Caregivers worth their weight in salt know the importance of slowing down. Savor your days off. Use them wisely. Take the time to see your life in reference to the bigger picture. Become aware of your own greatness.

TODAY: *Pause and reflect.*

Wise words from the psychologist Eric Frohm:

> Whether or not we are aware of it, there is nothing of which we are more ashamed than of not being ourselves and there is nothing that gives us greater pride and happiness than to think and to feel and to say what is ours.

We all have experienced the awkwardness of not being able to be ourselves around certain people. On some invisible level, the message is communicated that you must play along, pretend you are someone else or at least different than who you really are. In many instances, the other person wants you to be the way you used to be, your old self, before you got sober or married or had a baby or made whatever change you have made.

"Hey, you used to love my jokes, what's wrong?" they tease. "You're no fun anymore—you never want to party."

As we grow more clear and content with who we are, changes occur. More confident, we don't need the constant reassurance of groups to feel good. We don't need to escape with all-day shopping trips because we aren't afraid to be alone on a day off anymore.

People who don't or won't see our evolution are not interested in change. By not noticing who we have become, they don't have to think about who they are or have become.

You are not responsible for changing others or being someone you're not. If you've been pretending with another person, the time has come to stop. Does your spirit dim when you're together? Do you feel defensive or nervous? Pay attention to these physical cues that you aren't being authentic and be yourself. The world is waiting for you to be fully you; that is why you are here.

TODAY: *Be yourself.*

Television news reports bemoaned the circumstances and experts sounded the alarms:

> In recent years there has been a steady growth in the percentage of college men who are interested in computer science careers, but much less growth for women...Women's relative lack of computing confidence is likely to place them at a disadvantage when it comes to jobs.

Wait a minute; don't save this opinion to drive C so fast! The survey of new college freshman conducted each fall by UCLA's Education Research Institute compared student preferences in 1976 to the year 2000: the number of females interested in working with computers had risen from 1.4 percent to 1.8 percent of the 404,667 students tested. Among the males, the numbers had grown from 2.1 percent to 9.3 percent.

Since when do we measure a young person's readiness for employment based on his or her interest in sitting at a computer? Living in a nation where caregivers are in high demand but short supply, it seems we should be relieved by these numbers. Traditionally the gender that chooses to work with people, women continue to prefer animate over inanimate objects. The vulnerable infants and elders among us are eternally grateful that stalwart women obey the caregiving call. Why should this be a cause for concern?

> One of the most remarkable long-term reversals in the entire survey is that women continue to outpace men in their interest in a career as a physician," the report concluded, "this year seven percent of the women aspired to become physicians, compared with 4.8 percent of men. (Copyright 2001, USA TODAY. Reprinted with permission)

Our well-being as a people depends largely on how we treat one another. Indicators such as rising school killings, suicide rates, and incidents of child abuse reveal a nation that has less and less regard for life. Reading that technology has yet to woo away young women searching for a profession is good news, indeed.

More than ever, America needs to attract young people to the ancient and honored practice of caregiving. Computers have their place, and it isn't at the bedside.

TODAY: *Attract caregivers.*

Smoking is now linked to most of the leading causes of disease and death plaguing the Western world. Heart and lung disease, cancer and diabetes are all tied to cigarettes.

Caring for those ravaged by this nasty habit, smoking caregivers are certainly a living, coughing irony. In the United States, 25 percent of the over-18 population smokes, and in some nursing homes that figure is much higher.

My nonscientific observations have led me to conclude that very few Hispanic nursing home employees smoke. I have asked Spanish-speaking aides and nurses about this fact, and they have shrugged, saying, "It's not part of our culture."

How can we encourage non-smoking to be part of our nation's many other cultures? Research clearly indicates that women find it much harder to successfully quit smoking than men. I've known several men who decided to stop smoking and did so in one day, but know only one woman who has done the same.

Caregivers who suck smoke, knowing it is harmful, need our support and encouragement. Approaching the decision to quit, it is wise to frame one's plans using powerful, positive language. "Fighting" an addiction is exhausting and leads to more problems. The determined caregiver wisely focuses on his or her desire to be healthier, to breathe easier, with fewer chances for serious illness.

Marion repeatedly told her coworkers she was fighting the urge to smoke. Her cravings and weak willpower were her favorite subjects. She would launch into daily sermons on the mouth and how it missed its Marlboros.

Deciding to change their ways, smoking caregivers announce they are working on increasing their wellness and chances for a healthy old age, instead of dwelling on what they must give up. By choosing not to allow cigarettes a high profile, the smoker is far more likely to succeed at kicking the habit.

TODAY: *Choose health.*

Proud to be a CNA

I get up every morning at 5 AM
Don't think I'm not tired—I am! I am!
I take a shower and then do my hair
Put on a coat to fight the chill in the air.

Driving down the highway
Humming my favorite tunes
A smile on my face
I'll be at work soon!

What?! You don't believe it?
That my job makes me smile?
I love my work dearly
Every day I go the extra mile.

What is it that I do you say
That makes me feel so good?
My job is called a CNA—
Certified nurse's assistant to you.

—Devonna Lynn Bess

TODAY: *Be proud.*

Loving, compassionate people are part of every society. Like Detroit and other cities built on top of deep salt mines, civilizations are upheld by the presence of caregivers. Walter Trattner writes:

> The simplest method for aiding the poor, especially those unable to care for themselves, was for each family to care for a destitute person during a part of the year. ...the Hadley Town Meeting voted in 1687 that a certain widow should be sent, 'round the town,' to live two weeks with each family 'able to receive her.'

So dependent on husbands during this era of American history, women who were widowed were treated as homeless, helpless souls. Trattner continues:

> The most common seventeenth century practice, however was to place the poor in private homes at public expense. In some instances, the needy were maintained for long periods of time, up to 30 years and more. While this usually involved the payment of a fixed sum agreed upon for each person, with the town often supplying clothing and medical care besides, it was not unusual to auction off the needy...to the lowest bidder.

Imagine having no say in where or with whom you live for as many as 30 years of your life? The poor have always counted on the kindness of strangers, and as advanced as the world has become, the circumstances of the elderly poor have not changed all that much. An available bed is found by the hospital, and the frail Grandperson is transferred to your place of work.

Standing in the doorway, you greet the new resident and your life together begins. Bless you for being there, for being "able to receive her."

TODAY: *Receive new residents.*

(Reprinted with the permission of The Free Press, a Division of Simon & Schuster, Inc., from *From Poor Law to Welfare State: A History of Social Welfare in America* by Walter I. Trattner. Copyright © 1974, 1979, 1984, 1989 by The Free Press. Copyright © 1994, 1998 by Walter I. Trattner.)

How do you know if you are sugar-sensitive? Check each of the statements that applies:

1. I really like sweet foods.
2. I eat a lot of sweets.
3. I am very fond of bread, cereal, popcorn or pasta.
4. I now have or have had a problem with alcohol or drugs.
5. One or both of my parents are/were especially fond of sugar.
6. I am overweight and don't seem to be able to easily lose the extra pounds.
7. I continue to be depressed no matter what I do.
8. I often find myself overreacting to stress.
9. I have a history of anger that sometimes surprises even me.

If you checked three or more, find the book *Potatoes not Prozac* by Dr. Kathleen DesMaisons, as each of these statements relates to an aspect of sugar-sensitivity. The trick to feeling your best, according to Dr. DesMaisons, is to create a highly balanced system. For example, if you find yourself feeling impulsive and irritable, you are experiencing low serotonin. Have turkey for lunch. Three hours later have a complex-carbohydrate snack, like saltines or Triscuits. Or, referencing her book's title, eat Ole Mr. Spud at bedtime.

Be in service to your healing. If you feel grumpy and start drifting toward sugary things, go for a vigorous walk to raise your beta-endorphin level. If you feel muddy and unfocused, as if you're in a fog, eat some protein and get your body moving.

Living this way will give you confidence and awareness. Rather than being the victim of inherited body chemistry, you will find joy and delight in your sensitive and complex system. Your inquiring brain will find that food becomes fun and a powerful tool for feeling better and better.

TODAY: *Create a balanced system.*

Writer and home support worker Jodi Wilson of Alberta, Canada wrote this fictionalized story of her work:

> Margo is a home support worker. She has been coming for over a year now, and she has become quite fond of Mrs. Goldberg. Margo transfers her out of bed and takes her to the bathroom, where she helps her bathe. 'Oh, I can't tell you how good that warm water feels. You are an angel,' gushes Mrs. Goldberg.
>
> Margo gives her a hand putting on her clothes and getting herself moving. Mrs. Goldberg has arthritis, and it's Margo's job to help get her going in the morning. She chats with her while she prepares her a big of breakfast and realizes how much they both enjoy her visits. She is Mrs. Goldberg's link to the outside world, and she loves it. She says goodbye to her, and as Mrs. Goldberg smiles from the front window she feels a sense of truly having done something for someone.
>
> She has had a long day, and it hasn't been without its perks. She has managed to work eight hours and still make it to the theatre. She has brought some joy and a little conversation to an otherwise isolated woman. She has helped a man provide for his family and feel good about himself. Last, but not least, she has made sure someone got the right medication. Is her job important? Is her job rewarding? Is her job flexible? I think Margo, and every other Home Support Worker, would answer yes to all. The good news is a Home Support Worker can be a woman or a man and all cultures are required, one person reaching out and helping another.

By putting her thoughts and feelings on paper, nursing assistant Jodi Wilson was able to measure her job satisfaction for herself. If you're wondering whether caregiving is your life's work, follow Jodi's example and write a short story or essay, describing the rewards of the job. Listen to your own voice, and hear the song of the angels.

TODAY: *Write about job satisfaction.*

Valerie "Bull Star" Cooper, a CNA in Alabama explains her approach to writing:

> My poems are usually prayers to the Creator. Something just comes together and stays with me, helping me deal with a difficult situation. Many times the same things that are frustrating me are upsetting others around me. At first I was very reluctant to share things outside of my close friends and family. Then I realized that they were sharing it with others, and the poem came back to me, making a circle. When this happened several times, I opened up more and shared items more with those that I did not even have contact with directly. I believe lives change through sharing.
>
> An example of this is *A Prayer to the Creator*. It is all over the nursing home, in the break room, coworkers have taken it home and a number of residents' families have expressed enjoyment over it.

A Prayer to the Creator

> Give us Hope in our lives with our family and coworkers.
> Help me find the good in people's hearts and soul, not in the color of their skin or their actions.
> Let me be strong and good in each gathering in my life.
> Creator, give me the peace to ask forgiveness when needed.
> Give me strength and understanding for those who cross my path.
> Help me understand the needs of others, in this world and the world of the ancestors.
> Creator, help me to understand that with each difficulty comes growth of spirit.
> My walk on the red road of life will have rocks and sometimes boulders along the way, but I thank you, Creator, for being there always.

TODAY: *Change lives through sharing.*

Violations of human rights occur daily in nursing homes. During my national trips, nursing assistants share personal stories of poor treatment by management, where they have been publicly reprimanded, threatened or otherwise disrespected. Many confide the same painful observation: "We're the bottom of the barrel. The bottom of the totem pole."

I am frankly amazed that any human being, regardless of position or title, feels justified in verbally abusing another human being. When power and decision-making is centralized at the top, a skewed view of the world can hold hostage the otherwise good judgment and common sense of administrators. Feeling the pressure of being responsible for virtually everything, department heads may regard staff as the cause of problems and not the solution.

An aide's perception that s/he is the lowest of the low is partially true: the foundation is at the bottom. But being the foundation is not the same as being the least important; it is the single most critical determinant when sizing up an institution. Caregiving staff forms the basis for facility quality; without top performance, no amount of good management, nice wallpaper or excellent food can save the sinking ship.

Excellent healthcare institutions are built on a rock-solid foundation of reliable, compassionate caregivers. Regardless of changes in patients, management, the economy or even the weather, these Caregivers of Salt keep the world going 'round.

TODAY: *Be the foundation.*

I surveyed the staff of a large Massachusetts nursing home about their eating habits. Of the 100 respondents, only 15 ate breakfast. "I only eat one meal a day, after work." "I feel sick if I eat breakfast." "I get tired if I eat."

Instead of a meal, a large number of long-term care professionals drink soda pop for breakfast. And lunch. And dinner.

What are you putting into your body?

Author John Lee writes:

> One can of cola contains nine teaspoons of sugar. Dumping nine teaspoons of sugar into your body is a setup for wildly fluctuating blood sugar levels, weight gain, insulin resistance and adrenal fatigue, a perfect setup for hormone imbalance. Just as bad are the diet sodas with Nutrasweet, a synthetic chemical containing substances known to cause brain damage and may contribute to hyperactivity, learning disabilities and Alzheimer's.

In my ninth grade science class, Mr. Hollowell dropped a piece of roast beef into a bottle of coke. The next day, the meat had disappeared. "That's what will happen to your stomach," Mr. Hollowell told us. "Cola eats it away."

I may be one of the few people on the planet that has never consumed a can or bottle of Coke. Never. Beyond dissolving beef, what are the powers of cola?

In many states the highway patrol carries Coke to remove blood from the highway after accidents. Coke is also good for cleaning toilets, removing rust, cleaning corrosion from car battery terminals, haze from windshields and grease stains from clothes. Coke also kills laboratory rats, depletes the body of calcium, rots teeth, increases risk of yeast infections and makes you thirsty. Why not drink water instead?

In a University of Washington study, lack of water was identified as the number one trigger of daytime fatigue. Preliminary research indicates that 8 to 10 glasses of water a day could significantly ease back and joint pain for up to eighty percent of sufferers. A mere two percent drop in body water can trigger fuzzy short-term memory and trouble focusing.

Drinking five glasses of water daily decreases the risk of colon cancer by forty-five percent, can slash the risk of breast cancer by nearly eighty percent, and leaves one fifty percent less likely to develop bladder cancer. Are you drinking enough water?

TODAY: *Drink water.*

Renata's recipe for success as a nursing assistant at St. Patrick's Manor in Framingham, Massachusetts is part common sense and part magic, with a hefty pinch of salt added.

A gorgeous young woman with a 1,000-watt smile, Renata tells the story of one of her favorite residents—a very old woman who was totally blind.

"One morning I went in to get her up," Renata recalled. "She was crying softly about how much she missed the farm she had lived on all her life."

"'I miss the pigs and the chickens and the warm sunny days,'" she told me, "'Can you take me back to the farm, right now?'"

"I thought about what she needed because I wanted to bring her some peace. She was so upset," Renata said. Remembering the sunroom at the end of the hall, this resourceful caregiver made a decision. "I told her we would go for a walk, so she could get back to the farm. I brought her down to the sunroom, and I sat her in front of a window. The sun was pouring in. I opened the windows so she could feel and smell the breeze and listen to the sounds of the outdoors."

Perched in her sunny spot, the little lady became joyous. "Oh, it is so good to be back on the farm! The sun feels wonderful! Thank you!" she sang out. A few days later, the little lady fell, broke her hip and died suddenly.

"Just before she died, she told me her day on the farm was her happiest day ever," Renata said. "I always have felt good that I listened and helped her get back to the farm one last time."

TODAY: *Work a bit of magic.*

Ben was a handsome blond RN working in a California nursing home. "I don't think I can do this work much longer," the young man said. "I can't believe it, but sexual harassment is going to make me quit."

Being a male in the 95-percent-female world of long-term care is a challenge. With women living longer than men, most of the residents of facilities are female. Add to this mix the tradition that women choose nursing as a profession and we can begin to see Ben's dilemma.

For the second time in his career, Ben had been charged by a resident with expressing inappropriate sexual behavior! Everyone knew the resident was fiercely attracted to Ben, and had in fact been staging her own inappropriate passes and scenes with him. When he refused her flirtation, as gently as he could, the resident got furious and turned on Ben, filing her complaint.

Immediately laid off pending investigation of the allegation, Ben was without work. "You're guilty until proven innocent when this happens," he said. "I can't go through this again."

In the long-term care workplace, women do rule. Like the buffalo herds that once roamed the prairies, nursing homes are a matriarchal society!

What can we do to help the brave men who enter our kingdom? Be sensitive to their circumstances, and avoid off-color humor that isn't appreciated. Offer to work with them when possible, so they are not left alone with a female resident who might take advantage of the situation.

And don't ask them to lift all the time! Like stampeding buffalo, we end up driving these guys right out the building.

TODAY: *Assist male staff.*

Ludie Mae Jenkins is a certified nursing assistant in Georgia. Most of her kin are caregivers; even her grandson works in a care home. Hundreds of strangers have called Ludie Mae their favorite over the years, falling in love with her willingness to serve. During several decades of service, Ludie Mae has encountered few knots she couldn't untie. With Ludie's will, there's a way.

But a change in federal law finally caused this royal woman to stumble. "I've always come in on my days off to do special things for the residents," Ludie Mae explained. "Now they tell me it is against the rules to volunteer here. Just when am I supposed to do the extras?"

Concerned that dishonest employers might force caregivers to work off the clock, legislators implemented a regulation prohibiting staff from donating time in the facility. As with many government actions, this attempt to protect some hurts many others.

"Nobody is forcing me to come over here!" Ludie Mae said indignantly, upon hearing the reasoning that ended her days as a facility volunteer. "I want to be in here. I like coming in and fixing their hair and such."

Perhaps federal and state regulators didn't consider or imagine caregivers of such high standards existed. Far from feeling put upon or pushed, Ludie Mae views additional time in her facility as a blessing. Not worried about the time or schedules, she can enjoy the company of her residents at her own pace. What an extraordinarily good woman—a pillar.

Has Ludie Mae given up? "I am going to visit when I want, and if some government man has a problem with that, he can come see me."

Wouldn't we all like to be flies on the wall for that conversation?!

TODAY: *Enjoy the company of residents.*

In 2700 BC, more than 4700 years ago, the Chinese wrote of 40 different kinds of salt in the Peng-Tzao-Kan-Mu, probably the earliest known book on pharmacology.

Forty kinds of salt! Sounds like the personalities on the day shift! A diversity of strong-willed, good-hearted men and women make your facility a home. Evelyn's unique ability to get shy residents talking is as important as Mattie's gift at curing "bed-head" by fashioning pretty hairstyles.

But what about Deb and Janet and Helen, who've been aides for 28 and 25 and 44 years? Can we expect them to continue lifting and transferring tons of human beings every week? Can we design a special senior aide position for these old-timers, who need to reduce the wear and tear on their bodies?

Rather than losing the great wisdom and experience of veteran caregivers, facilities would be wise to offer promotions into teaching and training jobs. What about utilizing these gifted staff to handle paperwork, such as scheduling, inventory, and data collection for resident assessments?

Successful enterprises capitalize on the combined wisdom of faithful employees by continuing to involve them in daily operations. Start brainstorming now with coworkers, discovering ways to reduce the physical toll of caregiving. Hold onto experienced staff.

TODAY: *Keep veteran employees.*

For all our knowledge and skills, we human beings are a frightened bunch. Fear is a powerful motivator. Parents, teachers and bosses all count on fear to boost their ability to control others. Annual inspections of healthcare facilities are driven entirely by caregiver fear—fear of the dreaded deficiency.

In the motion picture world, entertainers and producers tap into our reservoirs of fear, knowing we have a love-hate relationship with the emotion. Yes, we hate to be frightened and yes, we love to be frightened.

Remembering the fun of a safe Halloween night, nursing homes are opening their doors to area families. Staff and residents work together to create spooky decorations and delicious treats. Noting the changes in public security that have made trick-or-treating a dangerous practice, caregivers have seized this new opportunity for the community to visit.

While a fear of aging or death, fueled by disturbing media reports, normally make many children and their parents afraid to enter a nursing facility, on the night known for the most fear they flock in!

Why not capitalize on this fateful twist, and create clever yet meaningful ways to connect with your visitors? How about handing them a scavenger list when they enter, directing them to:

Go see the retired town clerk of Glover—she's not far. Visit Miss Betty, and she'll give you a Snickers bar. Find the nurse aide wearing a crown; she's worked here 34 years. Get a goodie from Queen Alice; she'll take away all fears.
Sign our guest book as you go out the front door, and we'll invite you to the next community party we have in store!

Make up your own fun tasks that will introduce neighbors to the loving spirit of your home. On this scary night, let love outshine all fears.

TODAY: *Overcome fears.*

November: You are the light of the world.

A city set on a hill cannot be hidden. Nor do men light a lamp and put it under a bushel, but on the lamp stand; and it gives light to all who are in the house.

Who better knows the power of light than the late-night traveler lost on back country roads? A flickering kitchen window in the distance replaces fear with hope, confusion with direction.

You, too, are a beacon of hope and direction to all who cross your path. Radiating love, you have what the world wants, what all who are in the house seek.

Your light is so different from the neon lights of the dark streets, screaming *buy sell drink eat go.* Tied to none of these distractions, you possess an inner warmth and light that attracts others who seek to know the fire that burns within.

Caregivers of Light find identity and value in being true to the divine spark. Meaning and joy aren't found living in darkness, chasing the trappings and attachments of the world. You know greed and anger are the only prizes won pursuing material wealth.

In your shadow, others can be freed of victimizing compulsions that bring no peace. In your presence, they will turn from the flash of outside distractions and go inside to seek the illuminated soul. Casting Pure Light, you create an environment where others yearn for self-awareness.

Long before the time of Jesus' Transfiguration, when he blazed with bright light, great civilizations recognized this same light as the energy of life. In India, it is called Prana, the breath of life. The Chinese speak of universal energy as Ch'i. In Jewish mystical theology, the Kabbalah refers to astral light.

We look into your sparkling eyes and see you hold the same healing light within; it provides your power, certainty, compassion and patience. Your light is your message.

Prayer for Caregivers

>Source of Life,
>Spirit of All Healing,
>Bless those who
>Serve the sick.
>Direct and guide us.
>Remembering
>That each of us
>Will take our turns
>In darkness and in light,
>Let us be light
>For one another
>When the darkness falls.
>Gentle our hands.
>Soften our eyes.
>Open a window
>In our hearts
>So that Your Grace
>And loving kindness
>May shine through.
>Make of our attention
>A safe shelter
>For the healing
>Of the sick,
>In mind and heart,
>Spirit and body.
>Renew us always
>In Your love,
>Amen.

—Anonymous

TODAY: *Be light for one another.*

(Thanks to Pat McNeeley of the Little Sisters of the Poor in Warrensville Heights, Ohio, who created bookmarks for staff featuring the Christian version of this prayer. That version opens with "Christ Jesus.")

Anna is in her late fifties. She has been taking care of others since she has known herself. Now a diabetic with low resistance to colds and flu, Anna says she sometimes feels as frail as her patients. She has cut back on her hours in the nursing home so she can get enough rest.

"I want a story about me in the newspaper,"she announced to the facility administrator, "with a picture of me in my clean, pressed uniform."

"I've been taking care of people all my life, and I want others to know."

As children, we are taught such self-promotion is not appropriate, that we shouldn't "toot our own horns." Following this guidance, caregivers remain silent and polite, caring but not daring.

Meanwhile, the radio and television blast and blaze with news of schoolboy killers, family members who murder one another, and warring nations that can't make peace. Do we want to hear their horns exclusively?

The world is hungry for good news-for stories of loving, caring people like Anna. Few editors assign reporters to chase down uplifting events or occurrences. As a consequence, young people aren't introduced to caregiving as a possible profession. Why would anyone want to work as a caregiver when the reports only cover how you abuse, neglect and exploit the vulnerable?

Quality caregivers who have served others for many years must step up and tell their stories. American society needs to hear a caregiver symphony of tooting horns, playing your love songs about valuing life. Anna isn't being conceited or stuck up; she is a lifeguard, saving us from drowning in a sea of violent and negative news.

As a career caregiver, Anna has every reason to march down to the local newspaper and offer her life story as ripe for the writing. So do you. We can't afford your silence any longer.

TODAY: *Toot your horn!*

Benedictine Sister and author Joan Chittister writes, "Awareness of the sacred life is what holds our world together and the lack of awareness and sacred care is tearing it apart."

Sacred life is lived well beyond churches and monasteries. Wherever life is valued and regarded as precious and worthy of our respect, the setting is sacred.

Sherrie Barber, a certified nursing assistant in Anderson, Missouri, has always considered her work a privilege and honor. With a gentle touch, she works with residents without pushing or demanding. So considerate and sweet, Sherrie used to look like she was play-acting when she pulled out a cigarette and lit up.

How could this woman, who clearly sees the sacred all around her, be so unaware of her own holy nature? How could she willingly hurt her unique and beautiful self? Talking with other caregivers about her coughing fits and shortness of breath, Sherrie began to see her smoking as a symbol, an example of how she was not valuing life. In this light, smoking stopped being a pleasure and instead became another form of the pollution which was destroying her and the planet for her grandchildren.

Sister Joan Chittister continues:

> We have covered the earth with concrete and wonder why children have little respect for the land. We spill refuse into our rivers and wonder why boaters drop their paper plates and plastic bags and old shoes overboard. We pump pollution into our skies and question the rising incidence of lung cancer. We produce items that do not decay and package things in containers that cannot be recycled. We fill our foods with preservatives that poison the human body and wonder why we're not as well as we used to be. We make earth and heaven one large dump and wonder why whole species of animals are becoming extinct and forests have disappeared.

After 35 years of smoking, Sherrie made a decision: her life was sacred:

> I quit after attending a national nursing assistant leadership council retreat in September 1998. The council gave me the courage I needed and faith in myself to be a better person. I do believe that most CNAs are like me in that we have very low self-esteem maybe because we've always been put down....I really feel CNAs everywhere should be told how important they are, how vital they are to the elderly and the handicapped. CNAs are awesome!

Sherry lit her last cigarette, preferring to fan her inner light. Not long after she stopped smoking, she started learning about computers. Today, she owns a computer and is expanding her reach way beyond Anderson. " I never dreamed I could use a computer!" Sherry said. No longer spending on pollution, Sherrie has money to burn-on herself and her grandchildren.

TODAY: *See your life as sacred.*

Do miracles occur in modern times?

Theologians hold seminars and conferences to debate this question, but those who know Lolita Shepard, a nursing assistant in Arkansas, answer it with ease: "Absolutely!"

A single mother with an autistic son, Lolita cares at home and at work. Visitors to the Hamburg, Arkansas facility who want to meet this bright-eyed caregiver are told to "look for the woman with the welcoming smile." Dedicated to her profession and to developing her skills, Lolita is a member of statewide and national nurse aide associations. Between her books and the bedside, she learns daily about how to be a more skilled and competent care specialist.

"I believe we should always give a person a chance," Lolita said, explaining her attitude toward coworkers and residents. Approaching confusing or tense situations, Lolita's trusting, confident manner puts others at ease, making mountains into molehills. She avoids making snap decisions or judgments about people or circumstances, preferring to call upon her abiding love of others. Being in service, Lolita focuses on what is right for her resident, not on making herself right. In her care, frail elders learn they will be listened to and treated with dignity and respect.

When working with people labeled handicapped, Lolita believes the real disability lies within our hearts, as our fear stops us from loving. In her light, ruffled feathers are soothed and smiles return.

St. Augustine wrote, "Miracles do not happen in contradiction to nature, but only in contradiction to that which is known to us in nature." Lolita knows that all things are possible with love. With great openness and a spirit of generosity, Lolita makes miracles.

TODAY: *Make miracles.*

In northern Vermont, the sun is a welcome but infrequent visitor this time of year. On cold, gray days when light punches through the clouds, it is easy to see why native peoples worshiped a sun god. Source of light and warmth, the golden rays command our appreciation.

Not unlike the light that burns within, solar heat defines life. Both are embers of the divine, cheering us each day. Around the world, a constellation of mighty caregivers shines, stars that have devoted their lives to brightening the lives of others. Basking in a caregiver's love, the sick and needy of all ages feel cozy and secure.

Ever since my son was little, when we are not together at night we look for the moon: "Remember, that same moon shines on both of us!" We have always found great comfort in looking up.

Across all time zones, political persuasions and armed borders, light shines daily upon and within devoted caregivers. When tempted to feel gloomy, why not look instead toward the light? Link yourself to the men and women who stand as lamp posts in their communities, lighting the way for a more peaceful and loving planet.

A prayer written by nursing assistant Sue Tabron:

> May peace fill all the empty spaces around you,
> May contentment answer all your wishes.
> May comfort be yours, warm and soft like a sigh.
> And may the coming year show you that every day is
> really a first day, a new year.
> Let abundance be your constant companion, so that
> you have much to share.
> May mirth be near you always, like a lamp shining
> brightly on the many paths you travel.
> And remember that you are truly loved.

TODAY: *Look toward the light.*

Depending on how we measure a person's worth, one individual can be considered either a brilliant light or a sputtering flame. World history is generally taught by reciting the achievements of men in war and business. The contributions of women, raising one generation and burying another, are often overlooked.

Medieval witch-hunts were organized to suppress laywomen healers who served the peasant populations. Three hundred years of witch burnings were rooted in a mistrust of women's medical intuition, and the beginning of the ruling classes' campaign to put health care in the hands of highly-educated men only.

In their fascinating booklet *Witches, Midwives and Nurses, A History of Women Healers*, Barbara Ehrenreich and Deirdre English explain:

> The establishment of medicine as a profession, requiring university training, made it easy to bar women legally from practice. With few exceptions, the universities were closed to women, and licensing laws were established to prohibit all but university-trained doctors from practice...How did one particular set of healers, who happened to be male, white and middle class, manage to oust all the competing folk healers, midwives and other practitioners who had dominated the American medical scene in the 1800s?

The answer lies, according to professors Ehrenreich and English, in how the industrial giants who made their fortunes on oil and coal launched America's first large-scale charitable giving through the creation of foundations. Both the Rockefeller and Carnegie foundations opened during the first decade of the 20 th century, with reform of the medical profession a major goal.

The Popular Health Movement had many healthcare training programs and schools that readily accepted women students in fields that are still referred to as allied or alternative medicine today. Emphasis was placed on the patient knowing his or her body, on herbal remedies, a sound diet and common sense. But the Foundation men regarded this training as "irregular," and preferred the "regular" German-style medical university model, the first of which in the U.S. was Johns Hopkins, which opened in 1893.

Starting in 1903, foundation money began to pour into medical schools by the millions. The conditions were clear, conform to the Johns Hopkins model or close. The Carnegie Corporation sent Abraham Flexner on a national tour of medical schools. Flexner almost single-handedly decided who would get the money, and hence survive...The Flexner Report came out in 1910, and established medicine once and for all as a branch of higher learning, accessible only through lengthy and expensive university training. In its wake, medical schools closed by the score, including six of American's eight black medical schools and the majority of "irregu-lar" schools which had been a haven for female stu-dents...Doors were slammed shut to blacks, to the majority of women and to poor white men...Medicine had become a white, male, middle class occupation.

Looking across the ages, nurses and nursing assistants can better understand employment conditions today. Yes, in earlier times tremendous energy was devoted to hiding your cities of light, to placing a bushel over the lamp. But look again. Lights burn brightly in your workplace. Healing continues at the bedside; the lights have not gone out.

TODAY: *Understand history.*

Denise was one of the nurse aides who trained me. When her teenage son, Aaron, died trying to save his two nieces from a burning home, Denise said, "people say God will always give you enough strength to handle whatever comes, but this time, I don't know." Losing all three of these children, plus every picture and memento of her son, left Denise unimaginably low.

Friends and family rallied around her, but the loss was of epic proportions. Finding that everything in the community reminded her of death, Denise moved from Vermont to Texas, where she continues to work as an extraordinary nursing assistant. She says her faith has kept her from losing her mind.

Faith brings us superhuman power, giving us access to deep inner resources we may never have known. To find the energy needed to move across the nation, Denise searched her heart, where flickering coals inspired and guided her.

At a Massachusetts gathering of nursing assistants, we talked about high-stress moments that demand strong faith. Mary, of Malden, said that before entering a patient room on difficult days, she will say, "Thank you God for helping me. Amen." David, of West Newton, added, "If God doesn't help you, you can go crazy."

Turning inward for support, caregivers amaze themselves with the circumstances they can manage, the knots they can untangle. Joseph Chilton Pearce wrote, "To live a creative life, we must lose our fear of being wrong." The bright, shining light of faith drives fear out the fastest. With faith, creation occurs.

TODAY: *Turn inward for support.*

According to the U.S. Census Bureau, the fasting-growing segment of the population is currently those over one hundred years of age!

In his book *Live Long, Die Fast*, Dr. John Bland includes fascinating facts about aging:

> An unprecedented phenomenon is taking place: life expectancy for our species is rising....Life expectancy in the Middle Ages, from approximately 300 to 1000 A.D., was estimated to be about fifteen years; from 1000 to 1500 A.D. at about 20 years; from 1500 to 1700 at about thirty-five years; and as recently as 1900, life expectancy was about forty years. By 1993, however, life expectancy had risen to seventy-five years. By 2020, life expectancy should be more than double what it was in 1900— the greatest increase on recorded history.

What will define this longer life? Whom will it be spent with? Thinking one's old age will be less than what has preceded it, or more of the same, is reckless. The Italian composer Giuseppe Verdi, considered to have talent early in life, composed his last work, the opera Falstaff, when he was nearly 80 years old. After writing a series of popular tragic operas, Verdi surprised his fans when Falstaff premiered in Milan in 1893, as it was a comedy!

As caregivers, we have a sacred duty to know those in our care, to look past the disability and disease and into the depth of the soul. Together, your lights blend and fill the room, revealing what might have been invisible before.

"We often neglect the elderly, and in the process exclude them from the normal daily social experiences. This profoundly damages them," Dr. Bland writes. "In fact, isolation is a common cause of senility. Variety is not just the spice of life, it is the very stuff of it."

TODAY: *Illuminate the invisible.*

(From *Live Long, Die Fast: Playing the Aging Game to Win* by John H. Bland, M.D. Copyright © 1997 by John H. Bland, M.D. Reprinted by permission of Fairview Press.)

The Kabbalah is the Jewish book of mysticism and visions, truth and light. In the novel *The Book of Lights*, two young men, Gershon Loran and Arthur Leiden, read the Kabbalah as they study to become rabbis. Both men become chaplains during the Korean War. Leiden's only brother is killed, and then Leiden dies in a plane crash. Near the end of the book, Rabbi Gershon Loran has gone to see Dr. Malkuson, his professor of the Kabbalah, to seek solace and understanding. Why did a good man die? What is the point of life if such unfairness occurs? What can man believe in? Dr. Malkuson reflects:

> It is a great tragedy. The last of the sons. He looked down at the books. There was a long silence. Then he raised his eyes and directed his gaze at Gershon, and Gershon did not look away. 'I will tell you, Loran. What is of importance is not that there may be nothing. We have always acknowledged that as a possibility. What is important is that if indeed there is nothing, then we should be prepared to make something out of the only thing we have left to us—ourselves. I don't know what else to tell you, Loran. No one is in possession of all wisdom. No one.'

All caregivers have felt moments of such despair, when a beloved patient dies a painful death, or a coworker loses a child. Our lights dim; we wonder how we can go on.

Even the great wise professor shares this moment of doubt, and points us inside for answers. In the face of sorrow and injustice, reignite your light with the divine spark. Go deep inside and be warmed by the universal flame. Continue to radiate love.

TODAY: *Reignite your light.*

(Reprinted from *The Book of Lights* by Chaim Potok. New York, Fawcett Crest Books. Copyright © 1982, p. 383.)

How Do You Live Your Dash?

I met a man who stood to speak
At the funeral of a friend.
He referred to the dates on her tombstone
From the beginning...to the end.
He noted that first came her date of birth
And spoke the following date with tears,
But he said what mattered most of all
Was the dash between those years. (1934-1998)
For that dash represents all the time
That she spent alive on earth...
And now only those who loved her
Know what that little line is worth.
For it matters not, how much we own;
The cars...the house...the cash,
What matters is how we live and love
And how we spend our dash.
So think about this long and hard...
Are there things you'd like to change?
For you never know how much time is left,
That can still be rearranged.
If we could just slow down enough
To consider what's true and real,
And always try to understand
The way other people feel.
If we treat each other with respect,
And more often wear a smile..
Remembering that this special dash
Might only last a little while.
So, when your eulogy's being read
With your life's actions to rehash...
Would you be proud of the things they say
About how you spent your dash?

—Anonymous

TODAY: *Fully live your dash.*

I fall in love easily with CNAs.

For me, nursing assistants epitomize what is grand about being human: strangers can steal the hearts of strangers just by being themselves.

I fell head over heels in love with Arthur Coard, a CNA from Winter Haven, Florida, the moment we met at the Atlanta airport waiting for a shuttle. Was it his camouflage pants? His two pairs of purple glasses, one hooked on his overalls? Maybe all the body piercing or tattoos? Or the strawberry blonde ponytail?

Arthur was fully being himself, and it was so attractive. He hadn't settled on any standard, packaged look. Arthur knew what he liked and he wore his creativity well. His residents must absolutely adore seeing Art walk in each day. What will he look like today?

But beyond his glitz, Arthur's wonderful spirit, compassionate nature and easy laugh are the real draw. Because he is true to himself, Art's soul isn't in conflict. He isn't pretending to be someone he isn't.

Being with someone who is so open and genuine, I am invited to be myself. Arthur creates a safe harbor for others to express themselves. Arthur is himself, so I am myself, and then I encourage Arthur to be even more himself, and then he motivates me. Get the picture? When one is free to be oneself, experiences with others are deeply satisfying...for all parties.

Arthur confirmed my feelings with a recent card. He wrote on the envelope, next to my name, "My Motivator." Precisely what I call Arthur!

TODAY: *Motivate others by being yourself.*

When I was five years old, a happy day meant driving with my father to Jake's Bakery to get a powdered jelly donut. Like my dogs with their bones, I couldn't have been more content.

What does a happy day at work look like? Schedules are tight and everyone has more than enough to do, but what if you made the time to ask each other, "What do you want the day to look like?"

Getting this aerial view of the day, caregivers can shine their lights on the entire scene and see what's missing, what needs attention. Without such a pause you see only the narrow, dark confines of your hallway; your nose remains on the grindstone, and aching spirits can go unnoticed.

Tanya Looney of Alabama, a care specialist studying to be a nurse, turns to her residents for direction and inspiration, and writes poetry to share her awareness with colleagues:

When I walk on the hall,
I see a rainbow of faces,
A patchwork quilt with
So many stories to tell.
Weathered hands so soft
When they touch you,
Concerned about how our day goes,
Selfless and loving.
Our patients are our
Beacons of Light.
Helping us along our journey
Which is often dark.

TODAY: *Decide on the day.*

Certified more than 10 years, and having attended at least 12 hours of continuing education every year, America's nursing assistants are highly competent healthcare professionals. Nursing facilities and home health agencies that have survived tough economic times have done so, in large part, by listening to direct care workers. Helen Fisher writes:

> Even male business leaders no longer see the old hierarchical order as sacrosanct. To avoid what some call 'corporate Alzheimer's,'...and to attract capable staff, many have begun to believe that they must restructure their organizations. They are doing this by replacing the pyramidal command-and-control model with far more flexible, decentralized, less hierarchical office structures, as well as work units composed of team members who see themselves as coequals. (Reprinted from *The First Sex: The Natural Talents of Women and How They are Changing the World* by Helen Fisher. New York, Ballantine Books. Copyright © 1999 pp. 49-50.)

Consulting frontline staff on every patient decision is how healthcare enterprises will thrive in this millennium. Nursing assistants who provide primary care for a resident should be included in admission and roommate decisions, as well as regular meetings with physicians. Author Edgar Jackson advocates for a holistic approach:

> Already in many institutions a philosophy of patient care is emerging that considers needs in a broader perspective...The time seems ripe for changing the hierarchical structure and creating a value system based on what the team member can offer to patient care rather than personal status in the center's pecking order. (From *Understanding Health* by Edgar N. Jackson. SCM Press. Copyright © 1989.)

Closed meetings are no longer in anyone's best interest. Successful managers invite all involved parties to enlighten each other on patient care matters.

TODAY: *Enlighten.*

For many residents, the caregiver is truly the light at the end of the tunnel. Feeling guilty over-burdening exhausted family members, individuals in need of care sigh and cry at the sight of their capable caregiver. At last! Hands and hearts that know what do to and do it with great skill and tenderness.

Sick or not, all human beings seek the kind and loving interest of others. Regardless of our standing, we wonder if there isn't someone somewhere we need to meet, who has a message for us that will improve our lives.

Holy Mother Amritanandamayi, known as Holy Mother or Amma, is one of India's leading female lights, a spiritual leader to millions. Observers report that when she is with suffering and troubled people, "she absorbs their suffering and negativity into her own body. She blesses them and heals them with her gentle caresses."

So does Mary Sue Shane of Greenfield, Indiana. A loyal and able nursing assistant, Mary Sue took care of an overweight resident, "who cried and cried because she was so afraid when we tried to get her up." Working with her resident, Mary Sue gently introduced a new mechanical lift. With careful attention to her patient's needs, Mary Sue completed the transfer smoothly. "She cried and cried again, this time with joy, thanking me for her freedom!"

TODAY: *Heal with gentleness.*

We joke about married couples living together for so long they begin to physically resemble each other. The same can be said for partners at work.

Doris and Delores both work at Henning Healthcare Center in Henning, Minnesota. Like sisters, they dress alike, talk alike, wear their hair alike. Having worked together for years and years, they finish one another's sentences and each defers to the other with mutual respect. Coworkers count on Doris' and Delores' awesome stability, and joke that if the place is ever sold, this duo will remain, because "the fixtures stay!"

Given the intimate and demanding nature of caregiving, it is no surprise that coworkers bond so closely. We can't hide a bad day or the reason for it. Living with the same busy schedule and limited dollars, we trade tips on where to get a bargain on shoes or who does nails for less.

Sharing between caregivers is not limited to the visible. Perhaps even more easily conveyed are moods and attitudes. Of course Doris likes to work with Delores, and vice versa-they are both calm, kind, dependable women.

Will Archer retired after 20 years in the army and took a job as a nursing assistant in St. James, Missouri. Having worked in a predominantly male environment all his life, Will found the presence of female bonding and moods an unexpected education. "I've been married 23 years," he said, "But never understood my wife as well as the last three years I've worked in a nursing home!"

TODAY: *Enjoy your bonds.*

Caring deeply about the welfare and well-being of residents, caregivers are often frustrated by the lack of community involvement in their residents' lives. "We need more people to visit and listen," is a caregiver's common prayer, whether working in a healthcare institution or in a private home.

For a modest fee, a video is now available to show churches and other organizations different models for becoming involved in a healthcare ministry. *Labors of Love* is a 70-minute documentary on the many expressions of caring practiced in Minnesota by a variety of health ministries. A much shorter, inspirational version, *Health Ministries: A Universal Calling*, is also available.

Produced by the Minnesota chapter of the Health Ministries Association, the program was produced to stimulate discussion and encourage volunteers, and includes a study guide. Caregivers also share their experiences of serving rural elderly.

Among the topics presented are the importance of relationship and listening to well being, what it means to be "my neighbor's keeper," social justice issues and three major areas of particular concern to churches: peacekeeping, healthy choices for youth and guidance on end-of-life decisions.

Viewers are also introduced to the role of parish nurses as door-openers for those in need of advocacy or information about how to navigate the healthcare maze. Could you show the video at church or the next Family Council meeting? At your son's or daughter's school? Where can you attract volunteers with soul?

Order *Health Ministries: A Universal Calling* (5 minutes, $10) and *Labors of Love* (70 minutes, $15) from Laura Rydholm, Pastoral Care Immanuel St. Joseph's-Mayo Health System 1025 Marsh Street, Box 8673, Mankato, MN 56002-8673, rydholm.laura@mayo.edu, 507-389-4616.

TODAY: *Encourage volunteers with soul.*

Shake-ups shake us up. Management announces new turning schedules: "During meal times residents are to be on their backs, facing the window." "Who wrote this," the caregiver wonders, "someone who has never worked on the floor?" "Mealtimes have been left off the schedule completely so bedbound residents aren't even put in a position to eat!"

The beloved director of nursing who has served the facility for 18 years is put on an unspecified leave by the new owner: "Is he nuts? She's the best!"

Administrative ambushes are tough to handle. Without warning, a valued coworker is fired; a well-worn policy is replaced. Confidence in the decision-makers is shaky or worse. Those who "disappeared" are humiliated and lost; as one fired administrator put it, "I felt I had died."

Such times of upheaval require a sustaining inner light that provides caregivers with a focus, a sense of purpose and mission. Alliances with former staff members or procedures have evaporated, but one's connection to the source within must not waver. Grounded in a deep awareness of what is right and good, caregiver lights can survive gale-force winds.

A little English hymn is of great comfort when the weather inside is cloudy:

> We were born to shine with a pure, clear light
> Like a little candle, burning in the night
> In this world of darkness, so we must shine
> You in your small corner, and I in mine.

TODAY: *Remain a light.*

You Were Born To Shine

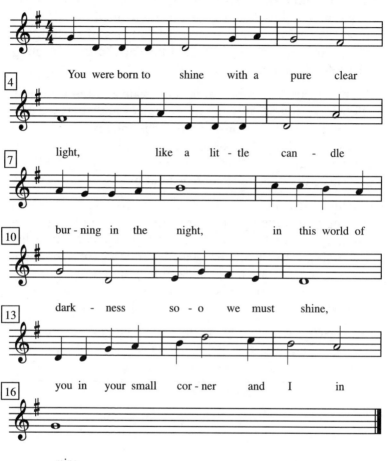

You were born to shine with a pure clear

light, like a lit - tle can - dle

bur - ning in the night, in this world of

dark - ness so - o we must shine,

you in your small cor - ner and I in

mine.

Author Carol Gilligan has studied the differences between the moral development of men and women, and discovered women define themselves in terms of their ability to care, while men value their rights and individuality: "Gilligan's more recent works aim to study the effects of such differences on work, and the effects of the social order on young girls' development."

From an early age most caregivers, male and female, value life and caring for it. How many nurses and aides tell stories of fixing their friends' broken dolls and rescuing injured birds? Of caring for an ailing grandmother or elderly neighbor when they were twelve years old? Like a tiny pilot light, the caregiver's desire to serve is lit at birth.

Phyllis Mitchell of Tekemah, Nebraska, has cared for others as long as anyone can remember. A certified nursing assistant, Phyllis applied to serve on a statewide care specialist leadership council, and needed a letter of recommendation. She shared her amazing story during a council meeting. "My first grade teacher is now my patient, so I asked her if she would write a reference for me," Phyllis grinned.

Her teacher wrote, "I knew Phyllis when she was six years old and she was a good girl then and is a good girl now. And she has always been well groomed!"

TODAY: *Honor your nature.*

My husband Thurmond is a musician, and he will tell you that musicians need listeners. Hearing him play the cello or sing, audience members find us after the concert and inevitably ask me, "Do you play an instrument?" I played the piano as a child, but it isn't a relationship I've nurtured as an adult.

"No, I'm a listener," I respond, and it's a responsibility I consider a great privilege. I love nothing more than having Thurmond play me a cello lullaby at bedtime. The give-and-take between performer and audience makes music what it is.

Like music making, caregiving also requires a twosome, a magical connection between parties. To be a healer, one must receive the gift of someone in need of healing. The late Methodist minister and healer Dr. Edgar N. Jackson was fascinated by these unseen links. He wrote:

> People who appear to have special endowments in aiding the healing process have been carefully studied. Dr. Lawrence LeShan has made such a study and reports these people all seem to share a common set of traits. As a group they tend to be warm, sensitive, loving people who approach others with utter selflessness. During the time when they are at work they appear to be in states of intense concentration.

Working as an aide, I witnessed this utter selflessness and intense concentration first-hand. While I was forever checking my watch to see why the morning had lasted 12 hours, the veteran staff, seasoned by years of experience, seemed to prefer a private, inner clock as a reference point. Like gardeners tending their plants, light-filled caregivers measure time moving from one resident to another. Straightening this, adjusting that, transferring him, lifting her; the passing day tick-tocks along in a series of satisfying moments. Suddenly, the shift ends. The joy, however, lasts.

TODAY: *Concentrate and connect.*

Our words can create darkness or light. The world's religions all emphasize right speech, as communication is considered a power that must be controlled in the spiritual life. In Buddhism, it is part of the Eightfold Path.

Christ taught his followers to avoid swearing, and to shun excessive and idle speech.

The Jewish doctrines stress the dangers of a wicked tongue.

Supporting the importance of choosing our words wisely, counselor Philip St. Romain wrote, "The quality of our relationships is largely determined by the manner in which we communicate, and not vice versa."

Our dog trainer insisted we never punish our puppy by using his name. "He'll come to think he is bad when he hears his name," she said. "To correct him, say 'bad dog' or 'no, doggie.'"

So from great spiritual leaders to pet teachers, there is agreement: our speech can bring sun or clouds. I come from a long line of talkers, and my son is carrying on the tradition!

I'm embarrassed to admit that he was terminated at his first job because of advice I gave him. Working in a nursing home kitchen, he was the morning dietary aide, delivering trays to the dining room and serving the residents.

"Honey, remember, you are the second person, after their aide, to greet these folks. Start the day out bright and cheerful! Talk with them."

When Elliot was fired, he was told he was a good employee, but he "talked too much to the residents." I strongly doubt that complaint came from the residents!

As a helping professional, finding the balance between conversation and action takes experience and example. Elliot didn't have either. Can you take a minute to help new folks find their way? Guide them in discovering what is too much or too little.

TODAY: *Speak lightly.*

In a roomful of 300 healthcare professionals I once asked, "How many people are mad at someone or believe someone is mad at them?"

Hands flew up, probably 150.

If asked the same question of a roomful of teachers, waitresses, repairman or saleswomen I am certain at least half would answer the same way. As human beings, managing anger and granting forgiveness are among our toughest assignments.

Unfinished business in this department keeps us awake at night. In the eighties, when I was having trouble sleeping, Dr. Scott Crandall told me the reason I couldn't sleep at night had something to do with what was happening during the day. Unfinished business.

Helping your patients get enough rest is a big portion of a caregiver's job. Besides making sure pillows are properly plumped and the blankets and room temperature in order, you often must minister to the subconscious—to the individual's soul. Assisting those who wake with nightmares and bad dreams requires careful attention.

Dr. Eric Dean, a professor at Wabash College in Wabash, Indiana, recommends that the reading of Psalms, if patients agree, would be quite a bit better for restless elders than sleeping pills or counting sheep! He suggests Psalms 4, 90 and 133 are wonderful words for putting someone in the mood for sleep. Like calming a child by reading a bedtime story, the creative caregiver may find a short Psalm is a balm. I practiced, and Psalm 4 takes less than a minute to read!

Use your own clarity and judgment to bring light to the night. Listen to unfinished business and apply a calming Psalm.

TODAY: *Help the sleepless.*

Remember those old spy movies, where in a pitch-black city, bad guys communicated by reflecting mirrors from tall buildings? Reflection is amazing.

Want more recognition for your contributions and good work? Look in the mirror.

Want to know who is responsible for whether today is a great day or a rotten day? Look in the mirror.

The face you shine on the world is reflected back many times over. And in the same mysterious way, you reflect back the faces you meet. How many times have you gone to work, your light flickering and dim like the weakened Tinkerbelle? Caught up in a funny remark or a resident's gratitude, your light begins to burn more bravely.

Mysteriously, another human being creates the right conditions for you to shine. You start the day anew.

Medical science has proven that the human body completely reproduces every cell every seven years. Like stating our age in dog years, we know that we are rejuvenated at age 7,14,21,28,35,42,49,56,63,70,77,84,91 and 98. At age 49, I am actually entering my seventh new skin, and am thrilled with the possibilities this brand new me presents. Deep within, the light of my faith continues to burn, inspiring me to be even more loving to myself and others. Stored pain of the past has been replaced with a clean slate.

Reflecting on yourself, look for ways you can begin anew today, re-dedicating your life to more fully being your true self.

TODAY: *Reflect.*

Alice Hersey is a soft-spoken, refined nursing assistant. A grandmother, her life and the goals she has set for herself demand lots of energy. Raising a grandbaby as well as working full-time, Alice is careful about adding one more responsibility to the day.

Yet upon watching another formula news story on the evils of nursing home life, this Mississippi care specialist decided she needed to extend her reach. She knew someone who knew someone who worked at the television station. Could Alice respond to some of the national stories being broadcast on the horrors of health care? Could they use her as an expert when nursing homes are in the news?

A filmed report is not the same as a live presentation, as it is difficult to capture spirit on tape. Alice's performance, however, glowed with truth and warmth. Speaking from the heart, she told viewers about the loving, safe community that flourishes at Broadmoor Healthcare in Meridian.

"Your face was glowing! You looked so beautiful on television!" staff and residents told Alice, and it was true. From her innermost source of compassion and strength, she found her voice.

So if you're keeping score, that's one point for the truth about nursing homes versus untold millions of points for the suspicious news media.

Alice is not a woman who looks for quick or easy solutions. Her life is about being a steady Christian soldier, marching onward with her message of kindness. She knows public opinion changes slowly. It took 30 years for the American consumer to begin questioning the popular message of cigarette companies: that smokers are cooler, have more fun and enjoy a better life.

Where can you bring truth and light? Is it time to extend your reach?

TODAY: *Extend your reach.*

During my son Elliot's thirteenth summer, we moved to the country, and he refused to come. After the usual wheedling on both sides, we agreed he could stay with the Friihaufs, another family in our old town, until school started.

Ed and Loretta Friihauf had fascinating careers and no children at home. A chemist-turned-innkeeper, Ed was now learning his third career, as a real estate appraiser. My cup of gratitude was running over when I dropped Elliot and his gear at their home.

"Bethany," Ed said earnestly, "do you really think, because you gave birth to this child, you are supposed to be able to meet his every need? Your job is help him get what he needs, but you aren't the only person he can learn from."

What a revelation! Mothers and fathers can ask for help? My guilt lifted like a cloud. Now a man, my son grew knowing many people loved and cared for him. I pass on Ed's wisdom knowing how many caregivers, especially single parents, are struggling to succeed in challenging healthcare careers while being attentive parents.

From within your ranks, many men and women are raising babies. Do you know who is caring for whom and what kind of special support they need? As busy as you are, time can be made to offer a little motherly advice or a promise to pray. Could you pick up a child after school, or pass along a good jacket your son has outgrown? Without overextending yourself, consult your heart and determine what you can offer.

TODAY: *Support children.*

I was married to Dr. Thurmond Knight on this day in 1990. We have both tried marriage before, wanting what a loving partnership and family can provide. We came together with a child apiece, and have spent the ensuing years creating that loving partnership and family.

Seeing pictures of couples celebrating their Golden Jubilee, I know we will be older than most when we hit that milestone. An impatient woman, I ask, "Do we have to wait? Why can't we take credit for time served in other marriages?"

With my fancy arithmetic, we will hold our 50th anniversary party in 2017! Having felt so outside the norm when I was divorced, the idea of publicly announcing this respectable achievement delights me.

Within your care there are dozens of individuals with similar stories and dreams, of divorces and widowhood, of abandonment and reconciliation. The budget for retirement parties was cut, and they never had a proper send-off. Children died or ran away, never to be heard from again.

We all have longings that fall short, prayers that went unanswered, and regrets that weigh us down. Your loving light casts a warm glow across the faces of those in your midst. Ask what anniversaries they wish they could celebrate, what parties they always had wanted. I heard about a single woman who told her friends she had been to 15 baby and wedding showers, and resented never being the center of attention. They decided to throw her an "it's about time" shower, and everyone had a ball.

In the spirit and name of love and healing, ask those you work with and care for what special holidays they would like to create and celebrate. How can you help them leave the darkness and bask in the light?

TODAY: *Create healing celebrations.*

Put me alone in a room with a Snickers bar, and I'll prove with great speed that humans are sensory beings. We relate to the world by tasting, touching, smelling, feeling, seeing and hearing.

Some of us are more trapped or controlled by our senses than others, as we struggle to juggle the latest diet, exercise plan and credit card offer. The world is forever whispering our names, tantalizing even the strongest among us with the latest new and improved temptation. When we meet someone who seems greater than their temptation, we want to know their secret.

"We are fascinated by people who are immune to the seductions of the physical world; they become our social and spiritual heroes."

Belinda is an absolutely gorgeous woman. Her flawless skin and flashing smile resemble the faces on the covers of *Vogue* and *People* magazines. A certified nursing assistant, Belinda's inner beauty radiates outward, causing all who see her to look twice or even three times.

"You are stunning," I said upon meeting Belinda. "Have you thought about modeling? You are a natural beauty!"

"Yes, I've been asked to model several times, and I've thought about it," she answered somewhat shyly. "But I've decided I want to do something meaningful with my life. I want to make a difference, and improve the lives of others."

Attending college part-time, Belinda wants to work for women's groups, to improve the conditions of women in the workplace. As a lobbyist, her beauty will get her appointments with decision-makers, and her message will be heard.

Combining her physical gifts with her deeper sense of purpose and meaning, Belinda has chosen a life of great depth and breadth. Each of us is called to integrate the human and divine within ourselves, and find a path that makes a difference and improves the lives of others.

TODAY: *Travel a meaningful path.*

With Hollywood and the nightly news providing so few "happy endings," it is truly uplifting to hear a tribute to quality caregivers. How often do we acknowledge the light-bearers for carrying the torch of kindness?

In October of 2000, I added my voice to the chorus of congratulations sung to Kathy Cote, Judy Deming and Penny Walker-Reen, considered heroines and lifesavers by the thousands of Vermonters they have served for a quarter of a century. Living in the small town of Morrisville, Vermont, these three sisters were honored by a county long-term care consortium, winning lifetime service awards. Kathy and Judy are both nurses who have worked at Copley Manor Nursing Home for more than 20 years—Kathy eventually as the administrator and Judy as director of nursing. Kathy's twin, Penny, has had the same tenure as an advocate for elders living in the community.

Few actions are as valued as providing comfort and housing to those in need. How many older Vermonters and their families have these sisters touched? How many individuals would lovingly speak the names of Kathy, Judy or Penny when telling their stories of facing personal moments of unwanted change or pain?

Working for the Central Vermont Council on Aging and later the Vermont Health Care Association over a 15-year period, I often crossed paths with these champions of the elderly. I have watched them humbly accept increased duties and promotions, never adorning themselves with the trappings of titles or power. Neither job descriptions nor hours in the week limit their responsiveness. Even in the days before pagers, you could find them and they would come.

When we are living near greatness, it is all too easy to regard it as the norm. Kathy, Judy and Penny's extraordinary, selfless model of community service is a standard few employees ever reach. The trio treats all who come to them as family, as worthy of their full attention, time and talents.

This is my toast to these three, which readers are encouraged to adapt and use to salute the light-bearers they work with:

There are angels among us
Tonight three sightings have been confirmed
God bless you Kathy, Judy and Penny
Through you, our faith in humanity is affirmed.

TODAY: *Salute the light-bearers.*

Thanksgiving is a time to express our gratitude for the blessings we enjoy, including the traditional bounteous meal of major comfort foods. Who could feel unfortunate with a plate of hot mashed potatoes and gravy in front of them?

When poor health and the need for 24-hour care enter our lives, appreciation may not come as easily. The whole Thanksgiving experience can become overwhelming, just like the mountain of food on the table.

Dividing the holiday into user-friendly pieces, caregivers can help patients celebrate in a manageable fashion. Sometimes the simple trick of serving the meal in several stages and portions helps the frail individual enjoy what would otherwise seem like too much to eat.

Thanksgiving week, hang paper tablecloths on the dining room walls at eye level, remembering eye level is lower for folks in wheelchairs. Provide crayons or markers and plenty of encouragement to "write down what you are grateful for!" Caregivers and residents alike are invited to add their thoughts: my children, my puppy, the garden, my eyesight improving. Giving thanks can be a wonderful personal and group exercise.

When the big meal is served, these decorated table coverings are placed on each table, further reminding all present that, indeed, there is much that makes us grateful. Taking a little extra time to focus on what we have, rather than what we have lost, is a loving way to observe the holiday.

TODAY: *Give thanks together.*

Debra Medders is a three-way bulb.

First click, she's a wife, mother, and grandmother. Stories of her family spill from Deb's lips and keyboard, overflowing with love and connection. Listeners have to figure out who everyone is: Kerry, Norie, Torie, Crystal.

Second click, Deb is a professional nursing assistant, concerned about residents getting a full day's worth of excellent attention, disinterested in excuses for why something was done poorly or not at all. Deb has created and led in-services on professionalism.

Third click, she's a writer. I don't think she realized she had this gift until a few years ago. I don't think she knew she had a third click in her. A desire to spread her light farther and brighter inspired Deb to begin to write.

She was in the middle of writing a book about the full life of a certified nursing assistant when another light bulb went off in her head: a children's book, *Peepy the Nursing Home Bird*. Based loosely on the antics of a pet bird in her Eupora, Mississippi facility, Peepy is a fast-paced story that teaches children that nursing homes are not places to fear.

As soon as she realized she needed an illustrator, an artist appeared in Debra's life, a volunteer at the facility. Now searching for a publisher for her beautiful story, three-click Debra Medders is planning other books and projects, expanding the portion of the world she lights up and calls home.

TODAY: *Find your next click.*

Anonymous acts are typically mean. My mother has always said that if I couldn't put my name to something, I wasn't to write it. I taught my son the same standard; if you don't want to be known as the author of a message, don't write or say anything.

But being around loving caregivers, I have learned there are also anonymous acts of kindness, wonderful moments when a word, a smile or gift is passed along, making my day a bit sweeter.

Following a presentation on seeing the extraordinary in the ordinary at the Avila Institute of Gerontology in Germantown, New York, a clear-eyed, confident woman came up to talk: "I have laryngitis, so I couldn't speak up during your talk. Have you read Longfellow's 'Psalm of Life?' I'm a CNA, and I live my life by it!" Her fervor was intense; I felt goose bumps rising on my arms. Goose bumps are always a good sign. They confirm I have just heard truth.

I said I had not read the poem, and promised to get a copy. Someone else began to talk and this beautiful stranger disappeared. I did not get her name, so I call her Every Woman, and thank her for introducing us all to Longfellow's directive.

A Psalm of Life

Tell me not in mournful numbers,
Life is but an empty dream!
For the soul is dead that slumbers,
And things are not what they seem.
Life is real! Life is earnest!
And the grave is not its goal;
Dust thou are, to dust thou returnest,
Was not spoken of the soul.
Not enjoyment, and not sorrow,
Is our destined end or way;
But to act, that each tomorrow
Find us farther than today.
Art is long, and Time is fleeting,

And our hearts, though stout and brave,
Still, like muffled drums, are beating
Funeral marches to the grave.
In the world's broad field of battle,
In the bivouac of Life,
Be not like dumb, driven cattle!
Be a hero in the strife!
Trust no Future, howe'er pleasant!
Let the dead Past bury its dead!
Act, act in the living Present!
Heart within, and God o'erhead!
Lives of great men all remind us
We can make our lives sublime,
And, departing, leave behind us
Footprints on the sand of time;
Footprints, that perhaps another,
Sailing o'er life's solemn main,
A forlorn and shipwrecked brother,
Seeing, shall take heart again.
Let us then be up and doing,
With a heart for any fate;
Still achieving, still pursuing,
Learn to labor and to wait.

TODAY: *Be a hero.*

December: Let your light shine before men in such a way that they may see your good works, and glorify your Father who is in heaven.

We see your good works in ever-widening circles of light, illuminating the lives of the world's Grandpersons.

In *The Zohar*, part of the Kabbalah—the Jewish book of mystical writings—it is written:

> There are lights upon lights, one more clear than another, each one dark by comparison with the one above it from which it receives its lights. As for the Supreme Cause, all lights are dark in its presence.

Faith-filled, trusting your instincts, you are Buddha and Mohammed and Jesus today:

—poor in spirit, answering a call, not rationally weighing career options. While the world may consider you powerless, humble caregivers enter each day with a deep sense of security and certainty.

—comforting mourners, forever making sacrifices and facing loss. Your challenge is to move others beyond the injustice, pain or cruelty, to accept and learn from sorrow.

—hard to rile or irritate, gently laughing off the annoying, seeing charm rather than harm.

—known for a positive attitude, reaching inside for strength and outside to serve. Having worked up a hunger to give, your personal peace comes through, obeying the call to love justice.

—merciful advocates for residents, not judging or applying conditions, but wanting for others what you want for yourselves.

—pure of heart, approaching work without needing a social reference. It matters not if a resident is a former janitor or a retired lawyer; each individual is welcomed as a blooming rose.

—peacemakers, because your single most driving desire is to assure and restore well-being. Conflicts are resolved before they escalate, as caregivers remain focused on returning everyone to this natural state.

—not looking to the world for affirmation or praise, you hold your head high. Far from being treated with regard, you may be falsely judged and cast off in favor of less principled workers.

—carriers of joy, responsible for spreading infectious laughter and giggles, breathing new life into old and tired attitudes. In the midst of gray sorrow, you affirm the uniqueness of individuals and celebrate life.

—seeking to preserve and improve, as salt preserves food from decay and corruption, you stabilize environments. In your salty presence, there is less upheaval and cutting of corners, for you are a deterrent.

—the presence of light, finding identity and value in being true to the divine spark.

When asked how she was feeling, my late friend Ruth Nims used to say, "I'm fine, except for this old lady business." Turning 90, Ruth suffered from ailments that kept her from doing much of what she loved. Occasionally a doctor would prescribe a bit of relief for her hiatal hernia, but most of the time Ruth had to live with various aches and limitations.

What helped Ruth the most were visits from family and friends. She kept her basket of Christmas cards next to her year-round; it gave her great pleasure to re-read newsy letters from former students and colleagues.

With ever-increasing technological advancements, some healthcare providers have become infatuated with wonder drugs and treatments. The term "sub-acute care" is especially hot, as doctors and nurses look for ways to improve or at least delay old age and its chronic companions.

The realistic patient like Ruth may find new, expensive techniques worth a try, but isn't fooled into expecting much. As my Dad says about his arthritis pain, "It only aches when I'm awake."

Holding out for the latest medical miracle is a common human trait. King Edward II's physician, who had a PhD from Oxford, convinced patients they would be cured of a toothache by writing on their jaw, "in the name of the father, the son and the Holy Ghost." His backup plan involved touching a needle to a caterpillar and then to the tooth!

Other remedies popular in earlier eras:

—to treat leprosy, a broth was made of the flesh of a black snake caught in a dry land among stones.

—dentistry routinely included taking the teeth of the hired help, like the stable boy, and implanting them into the gums of the lady of the house, so she had nice white teeth. Practiced with no painkillers, the implant was replaced every six weeks.

—Dr. F. Hollick, speaking of methods for curing a lack of menstrual periods, commented: "Some authors speak very highly of the good effects of leeches, applied to the genitals, a few days before the period is expected."

High-quality caregivers are open to new technology, but don't elevate it to a sacred place. More than being tethered to machines or dependent on expensive pills, patients want your time and touch. When prescribing care for the frail and infirm, contact with others is still the best medicine.

TODAY: *Touch.*

In the years I served nursing home residents as a long-term care ombudsman, I always loved an excuse to visit little St. Jude's Nursing Home in South Barre, Vermont. With around 30 residents, the renovated farmhouse was the homiest of institutions. But besides the comfortable old building, what made St. Jude's so wonderful was the director of nursing, Nancy Butryman.

Once I recognized Nancy was the heart of the operation, I would joke that the sign out front should read, "St. Butryman's." Nancy supervised the care of many challenging patients, some discharged to St. Jude's after a lifetime of living in the state medical hospital. Year after year, the home just chugged along, celebrating holidays and birthdays, welcoming volunteers and visitors. And no one died.

We know death is an ever-growing part of being in the long-term care business. Nursing homes are rapidly replacing hospitals as a final resting place. But not St. Jude's. Nancy's nurses and aides tended to their tiny flock like mother hens to their chicks. Nothing was overlooked.

I remember a male patient who had blown his eyes out in a hunting accident. His large, open head wound would not heal. Whenever I stopped by the home, almost always unannounced, it appeared the gentleman's dressing had just been changed.

Sister Joan Chittister's words about the meaning of work convey the philosophy Nancy Butryman instilled in all staff:

> Work develops the worker. The fact of the matter is that work is the one exercise in giving that always comes back to the giver. The more I work at anything, the better I get at it. And the better I get at something, the better I feel about myself. Work is the way I am saved from total self-centeredness. It gives me a reason to exist that is larger than myself. It makes me part of possibility. It gives me hope.

When economics forced the closure of St. Jude's, Nancy oversaw every patient's transfer and placement, and visited them in their new homes. Her deep sorrow over the break-up of her "family" was painful for all to witness, because her love for her patients was so authentic and abiding.

There will come a moment in life when we will have to ask ourselves what we spent our lives on and how life in general was better as a result of it. On that day we will know the sanctifying value of work.

Nancy need not fear that day of reckoning.

TODAY: *Love like family.*

Professional long-term care providers working in America today are standing upon a great threshold. The root word "thresh" means to beat out corn or grain, separating food from the unwanted, useless chaff. People once threshed wheat and other grains by placing stalks on frequently-traveled paths, such as the bottom of doorways, to efficiently harvest food just by walking about.

When I was in India, I saw many women placing armfuls of rice plants on the roadways in front of their homes so passing traffic would help with threshing.

As CNAs traveling the halls, you are mentally threshing out the useful from the useless aspects of day-to-day operations. By simply moving through the day, you know the scope of what CNAs can do. You have thrown out the useless identity of being an unskilled worker and found your kernel of truth: you are a vital and valued servant of our nation's aged and infirm.

A decade ago, nursing assistants needed daily direction and supervision from nurses. The idea of a nursing assistant serving on a care planning committee or handling the assignment of roommates was unheard of. Now, such responsibility and authority is essential to the healthy operation of a nursing home.

Your scope of practice includes ministering to troubled family members, inspiring discouraged patients and observing changes in behavior and conditions. Once employees who simply carried out the requests of others, nursing assistants have evolved into self-motivated, self-starting healers.

Has management noticed your transformation? Maybe. To be fair, managers have become more burdened by paperwork. CNAs were once the pack mules of the facility, with little freedom to create. Management is now saddled with this identity, with fewer and fewer opportunities to be creative and thoughtful.

TODAY: *Notice your growth.*

The first paperback book was published in 1933: *Lost Horizon*, the classic tale of an enchanted Shangri-La. Conway, the great adventurer in the novel, has lived a life full of death-defying activity. Reflecting on his latest predicament, he says:

> If you'd had all the experiences I've had, you'd know that there are times in life when the most comfortable thing to do is to nothing at all. Things happen to you and you just let them happen.

Few individuals know this truth as well as the experienced caregiver. How often cruel words are expressed by frustrated patients or coworkers-words that demand a response in kind.

"Don't talk to me right now," a nursing home maintenance director once said to me, "I'm counting to 1,000!" A wise man, he wasn't going to add to the morning's latest problem.

Timing is everything, both for knowing when to do something and for knowing when to do nothing at all. In this work for a few years, you begin to see cycles and patterns. Bob blows his stack on bath day. Deanna snaps the day before payday. Recognizing the rhythm of life in your workplace, you learn to function without being buffeted by changing conditions.

I'm an avid reader, and I used to worry when suddenly I didn't feel like reading one more word. My books are my best friends; was I abandoning them? I confided this fear to a caregiver friend, and she sounded like Conway himself: "Don't get all bent out of shape, Bethany! It will pass. In the meantime, today is your book—read it."

TODAY: *Let things happen.*

"They must have served beans last night!" Day shift caregivers know these mornings well, when it seems there aren't enough washcloths in the building. A few good jokes get passed around and everyone gets through it.

Chili is just one of the waves that can hit the building with force. Sometimes a visiting Boy Scout troop sets people off, increasing the noise levels on all floors. News of an impending storm or heat wave can have the same effect, putting even the calmest people on edge.

Is there a scientific explanation for these group mood swings? Is something bubbling under the surface?

As a matter of fact, yes. In 1964, physicist J. S. Bell published a mathematical proof called Bell's theorem. Bell's theorem supports the concept that subatomic "particles" are connected in some way that transcends space and time, so that anything that happens to one particle affects the other particles immediately. In Bell's theorem, effects can be "superluminal," or faster than the speed of light.

So what happens in room 110 between two unhappy roommates is experienced on some level at the same time in room 224. Surveillance cameras and gossips can't equal this instant, facility-wide broadcast!

You've always said you feel something "in your bones," and now you know why. Like any living organism, your facility has a pulse. Under one roof, you breathe and move together, dependent on one another for things great and small. Be mindful of your connections, knowing that what you say or do to one person influences all.

TODAY: *Be mindful of connections.*

A CNA from New York told me about the death of one of her patients:

> She was dying, and all she kept asking us was 'where's my purse?' We would reassure her constantly that it was tucked by her side, sometimes holding it up and pointing to it. After she died, we collected all her things. Someone looked in the purse. She had $700 in cash. I think she thought she could take it with her!

Believing we can somehow take our worldly goods with us into the next world is just one of mankind's well-worn mortality myths. No one was more prepared for this possibility than the royal families of ancient Egypt, who buried their mummified loves ones with food and riches.

Within the long-term care world, we frequently hear families say, "if you have home health you won't die, but if you move to a nursing home, you will."

I suspect this romantic view of home health is largely driven by the media. Frightening stories of poor care and premature death are ten or twenty times more frequently reported about nursing homes than about home health providers.

In truth, more people die at the hospital than at home or in the nursing home.

Unless your residents have worked in health care, funeral homes or come from an open, forthright family, it is doubtful they have had any meaningful conversations about death. Because you are comfortable with the subject, you create the safe space many need to talk about their end times. Promise yourself that if a resident, their family member or a coworker begins to share death worries, you will listen carefully. The sensitive nature of such discussions makes humor a tempting way out. Don't take it.

TODAY: *Listen for death worries.*

The regional personnel manager for a large nursing home group, Joey hears plenty of complaints. Among the most common problems reported to him involve unhappy family members. "No matter what we do for their loved one, it is never enough. 'Too little, too late,' that's how we're treated," he said. "What can we tell complaining families?"

Being clear, up-front and consistent with families about what they can expect from the facility is very smart. No, the CNAs will not be able to make their angry, stubborn, unhappy mother turn into a little lamb. No, we will not transform Dad the Hermit into Dad the Social Bug. We'll try—that's it.

Encourage family to talk about their fears. Sometimes people just need is to be heard; deep down they know there is no magic fairy dust you can spray around the room. Offer facilitated family council meetings where such fears and frustrations can be vented.

In helping staff handle belligerent, demanding and dissatisfied families, stress the saving grace of "not taking anything personally." Most families' frustrations predate the nursing home move. Address what you can, and regard the other rantings as the release of steam.

Sometimes family members feel powerless and guilty, and complaining temporarily masks these suffocating emotions. I once heard of a woman dying of end-stage cancer who refused to acknowledge her condition. "I feel so tired; it must be the flu," she told her caregivers on the day she died.

She refused all visits from her young children, claiming she didn't want them to "catch anything."

Such denial is tragic to witness, particularly for the competent, compassionate caregiver. In such circumstances, remember everyone has his or her own path. No one's life, or death, is like anyone else's. Be present, be loving, and do your best. The rest is out of your hands.

TODAY: *Understand troubled families.*

When I'm on the right track with a project or thought, my stomach offers me a zinging squeeze of vibrating confirmation. Hearing an especially powerful story of caregiving, I get goose bumps.

The great scientist Albert Einstein said he could tell he was on the right track by a tingling at the end of his fingers.

Trusting your gut is neither a new nor a foolish phenomenon. Though Western medicine may be slow to accept the obvious, our minds and body are not separate. The studies linking mental with physical health number in the thousands, begging the question, "Why do we see ourselves as two separate beings?"

Whether listening to ourselves or to others, our bodies are accurate little lie detectors. "Sure, I'll work on my day off," you tell the scheduler with a smile, while your stomach ties itself into a square knot. "Glad to meet you," your blind date winks, a trembling voice betraying his artificial self-confidence.

Phyllis knew something was wrong with Mrs. O'Brien. "Her vitals are fine," the charge nurse declared, "so she's fine." But having cared for Mrs. O'Brien for nearly three years, Phyllis had a sixth sense, an intuition that was loud and clear: something is wrong.

Elderly patients are especially vulnerable to this dismissive treatment-after all, "you're old, what do you expect?" What we all expect is that our caregivers will get to know us and our conditions.

Because her nurse aide remained firm that Mrs. O'Brien needed further attention, a diagnosis of depression brought on by a magnesium deficiency was made. Trusting her instincts, Phyllis carried out her duties in a highly professional manner.

TODAY: *Trust your gut.*

Sally can't bear silence. A bright and talented woman, Sally panics if she is riding in the elevator with someone and conversation stops. Revved up by nervous energy, she begins talking about this or that with great gusto, sometimes blurting out the craziest comments.

Firemen and other rescue personnel know that the adrenaline released during times of great stress is a wonderful propellant. Crises not only bring out the best in some people, they bring out the most. Looking back on his or her performance at an accident scene, an EMT can marvel at the stamina displayed. "I don't know how I held it all together," they reflect.

But fear of a lull in the conversation is not the same as encountering a five-car pileup at rush hour. One deserves little or none of our attention, while the other requires we pull out all the stops.

Unbridled nervous energy wears out the Sallys of the world, and all those within the sound of their voice. How many times can anyone hear repeated, "I sure hope we have a good summer. A good summer would sure be nice. Wouldn't you like a good summer?"

Exhausting to the speaker, the fumes emitted by a nervous person smother listeners. Be on the alert for times when your own speech is driven by anxiety, for moments when you are talking just to fill an empty space.

Take a deep breath. Cross your arms and give yourself a reassuring squeeze. Silence is okay! And if you hear Sally, or one of her sound-alikes, give her a hug, too.

TODAY: *Resist nervous chatter.*

This time of year in Vermont, we are becoming experts at tending our woodstoves. Starting the car on cold mornings is our second full-time job. Lest you Southerners think this means, "open the door, throw in wood," or "call the auto club," let me assure you that surviving a northern New England winter is an art and a science. I will forgo all the speeches about the type, size and age of the wood-that's an in-service unto itself. I will also omit the classic sermons on the importance of new car batteries and garage doors that close. Instead, I will dwell only on the critical fuel-to-air ratio.

When starting a cold stove, one needs more air rushing in than usual. When starting a cold engine, more fuel is needed than usual.

As each contraption warms up, we continue to adjust the air and the fuel. Watching the fire catch in the stove, we add bigger pieces of wood and close down the drafts and damper. Started properly, a successful wood stove fire burns slow and hot.

Once the car engine is warm, we can let up on the gas pedal. In the old trucks, the amount of air mixing with the gas is reduced or cut off with the choke. Once the engine is warm, there is no reason to choke off the air, so the choke is disengaged.

Finding these delicate balances of fuel to air is also important in our relationships with others. When we are new on the job, we need more help and people around us, giving us fuel: support and their wisdom. As we get more comfortable and certain, we can have more space, more air.

The perfect mixture for optimum performance is different for every stove, engine and person. To do our best and enjoy the day, we all need a mixture of assistance and independence, group and solo work. Pay attention to creating good conditions for yourself and others. Without them, we choke and sputter, unable to warm up and go.

TODAY: *Find balance.*

Facilities are like families, both with their own unique if not peculiar ways. I remember hearing nursing assistants talk about "doing their cares," in Minnesota, and "doing our run," in California. Both were referring to the personal care provided to patients in the morning.

Regardless of size or location, nursing homes have distinct approaches for handling the demands of day-to-day life, from how the mail gets distributed to whether disposable or cloth diapers are used. Working in one facility and moving to another, caregivers can be in for a few jolts, as they must learn new routines and practices.

The traditions of households and institutions are carried out by people. Listening to staff describe how or why an assignment is completed, we hear echoes of the past, the voices of loyal old-timers who built the roads now traveled.

In nature, this same phenomena appears, where a message repeats and repeats. Have you noticed that a twig has the shape of the branch it sprouts from and the branch has the shape of the tree?

According to researcher Benoit Mandelbrot that's only the start of the surprise.

Imagine the jagged coastline of Maine from a satellite view. Now picture zooming in on a bay. At this smaller scale the jaggedness reappears. Zoom in further to a stretch along one side of the bay and jagged sub-bays appear. Mandelbrot says we can continue to zoom all the way down to the grains of rock and sand and the self-similarity will continually reappear.

Life, however unpredictable and difficult, is not an accident. Between sunrise and sunset many repeating images of beauty and majesty occur. Caregivers are privileged to work on an exciting stage, where comedy and tragedy play daily. Take comfort in the tried and true traditions around you; see yourself as a perpetuating a proven high standard.

TODAY: *Perpetuate high standards.*

Nurses say thank you.

CNAs are very loving people. They cuddle and love the residents and brag about their residents. I don't always get the chance to thank the aides before they leave. So let me say, 'Thank you!' for all the hard work and loving care you give. Many CNAs entertain their residents as they care for them. For instance, they sing to residents, make them smile and even laugh.

Thank you for:

Accepting sudden changes of assignments
Anticipating not only resident needs, but nurses' needs
Arriving on time
Leaving things in order as you leave your shift
Realizing many residents you attend cannot express gratitude
Treating the residents as if they were family members
Informing the nurse of changes in condition
Offering drinks to the thirsty
Accepting unpredictable short-staffing situations
Welcoming new workers
Exhibiting a humble attitude
Attending to routine chores without being asked
Taking charge when a nurse must leave the unit or attend to the critically ill
Accurately maintaining records, including I and Os
Spending that extra minute to comb someone's untidy hair
Listening to repetitive stories with interest
Treating all with dignity

—St. Patrick's Residence, Naperville, Illinois

TODAY: *Feel appreciated.*

Caregiving is practiced on several levels simultaneously. To minister to the whole patient, caregivers must be aware of both their care and cure energies.

Caring is regarded as female, or in the Chinese tradition, the Yin energy. Rooted in an inner reality, caring relies upon intuition, wisdom and understanding. Relationship is of utmost importance when caring, and creates an active sense of belonging and connectedness. Caring providers are highly receptive to what the patient needs and are aware of unseen needs.

Curing is regarded as male, or in the Chinese tradition, the Yang energy. Focused on curing, the provider maintains objectivity. Emphasis is placed on knowledge, reason and linear thinking. The curegiver works to master the facts surrounding the visible needs, observations which direct his or her actions. Unlike those with a care orientation, those based in a cure foundation see themselves as separate and apart from the patient.

Emily knew Edgar Johnson was dying of lung cancer. But she also knew that his infected toenails were the source of great pain and preoccupation. Working the doctor, Emily helped Edgar heal his feet so walking was no longer an excruciating experience. As Edgar soaked his feet and Emily applied ointment, they enjoyed some good conversations about Edgar's life as a highway engineer. Utilizing a blend of curing and caring, Emily was able to serve her patient on the seen and unseen levels of his needs.

TODAY: *Blend care and cure.*

Marion lives a few miles from the Canadian border. Scheduled as the guest speaker at a women's club, Marion received a call that the meeting location had changed. "We have more registrations than usual, so we needed a bigger place. We're going to meet at a bigger home in Rock Island."

Almost visible from the Vermont side of the border, Rock Island is in Quebec, about 10 miles from Marion's house. "I'm an international speaker now!" Marion announced with a laugh, following her Canadian appearance.

All joking aside, Marion knows the power of labels, of giving oneself headlines to live under. Billing herself as an international speaker, Marion lifted her own expectations and standards. She tapped into the extraordinary energy of language.

I read of a parochial school, where the principal felt teachers had started to lose some of their zeal. Unlike the public school staff, the faculty at this church-sponsored elementary were supposed to teach the core curriculum plus Christian values. Over time, the religious training had taken a backseat, and the principal wanted to revitalize the teachers' commitment.

Over the weekend, he hung signs above the doorways to each classroom: "You are now entering mission land." During a follow-up discussion during the weekly staff meeting, the teachers said they had taken the reminder to heart.

In the first 1,000 years of Christianity, health care provided outside the family was the responsibility of the Church. A sign was placed upon the door of infirmaries and hospices: "The greater the victim's misery, the greater the attendant's value and merit."

In today's healthcare institutions, this ancient infirmary sign still holds true. The more difficult and demanding a patient, the more critical the caregiver becomes. Taking care of a light care resident is one thing. Serving a heavy care resident needing skilled nursing is quite another.

Have you thought about what kind of sign should hang over your wing? Knowing the power of words and the history of infirmary signs, "A" or "B" Wing hardly seems adequate. Share your thoughts with others, and consider placing signs in your facility that speak to the holy nature of your privileged work.

TODAY: *Hang a sign.*

Government is forever mandating a new law or regulation designed to make life better, safer, or fairer. At this writing, adequate nurse staffing in nursing homes is the subject of newly-introduced federal legislation. HR 5646 would direct state inspectors to examine the roles that staffing shortages play in causing harm to residents. If a lack of nursing coverage is found to be a contributing factor, facilities would be given 30 days to hire the additional nursing staff necessary to assure resident well-being.

Responding to calls for mandatory staffing ratios, the National Association of Geriatric Nursing Assistants (NAGNA) has gone on the record saying:

> You can pass laws, but you can't do magic. There is no unwillingness to hire CNAs; we just don't have qualified applicants! Mandating ratios would only result in surveyors writing staffing deficiencies in every facility across the nation.

NAGNA estimates nationwide there are currently an average of seven CNA openings per facility.

The proposed legislation is apparently based on the "build it and they will come" philosophy. Beyond the shortsightedness of thinking that a law will attract more individuals to a career in long-term care, such legislation is also flawed in assuming a fixed number of nurses and aides are right for all circumstances. As any parent in a large family knows, more one-on-one attention is required on some days than on others. Depending on the needs of patients, the complement of nursing staff can range quite dramatically.

Rather than demanding providers hire staff who don't exist, why doesn't the government launch a major recruiting campaign with providers, to attract new caregivers to the field?

In helping providers improve their image the government can do more to improve care than it would in mandating staffing levels or leveling fines. Please, Congress, get off the providers' backs and stand by our side.

TODAY: *Tell your story.*

McGill Cancer Center scientists surveyed 118 oncologists who specialized in the treatment of lung cancer. The physicians were asked what they would do if they developed the disease. Remarkably, three-quarters said they would not participate in any of the current chemotherapy trials.

Why? Because they considered chemotherapy ineffective and poisonous:

> An analysis of the study discovered that the more familiar physicians were with the particular forms of chemotherapy, the less willing they were to undergo them. In 1989, 150 oncologists at research units around the world were surveyed about the cancer treatment choices they would make for themselves. With alarmingly regularity, oncologists say that they would not allow chemotherapy to be given either to themselves or to their families. (From the book *Reclaiming Our Health*. Copyright © 1996, 1998 by John Robbins. Reprinted with permission of H J Kramer/New World Library, Novato, CA. www.newworldlibrary.com or 800-972-6657 ext. 52.)

Where does "Do Unto Others" fit in here?

Assessing the strengths and weaknesses of your facility, would you suggest a family member move in?

Caregivers can participate in all kinds of fancy job satisfaction surveys and workshops, but the key question is, "Is this place good enough for you and your family?"

If not, commit yourself today to do what needs to be done to make it good enough. Is management tuned out? Are the frontline staff lazy or depressed? Is patient privacy missing in action?

Completing all their studies and exams, doctors pledge to do no harm and say the Hippocratic Oath. Not the hypocrite's oath. Make sure you are clear what Oath you live by, as well.

TODAY: *Support your facility.*

Caring for individuals suffering with Alzheimer's in a private home is next to impossible. Regular household conveniences and appliances become weapons of destruction and death. A simple stairway is a life-threatening hazard. Regardless of a family's passion or resolve, few can manage to care for a loved one with Alzheimer's at home. Exhausted and discouraged, most families turn to a nursing home or other residential care setting for help.

Historically, institutions have been built for just these kinds of circumstances, to meet the unmet needs of the community. In 1908, the International Congress on Tuberculosis produced several significant papers that emphasized the futility of home treatment for patients with TB.

Most important was a paper read by Dr. Arthur Newsholme, an expert on vital statistics. Newsholme showed the tuberculosis death rate was directly linked to the quality of hospital or institutional care. Not only was care better, but with carriers removed from the home, the infection rate dropped dramatically.

Many reformers left the Congress convinced that, both on humanitarian grounds and in the interest of public safety, no substitute could be found for institutional care.

Immediately following this medical meeting, tuberculosis sanitariums were funded by government and built across the country. Far from considering the move from the private home to an institution cause for alarm, families and patients recognized their good fortune.

Remember the value of the service you provide, especially when families seem upset to have admitted their mom or dad into the facility. Emotions aside, they would probably acknowledge great relief in knowing that you are there.

TODAY: *See the role of institutions.*

(Reprinted with the permission of The Free Press, a Division of Simon & Schuster, Inc., from *From Poor Law to Welfare State: A History of Social Welfare in America* by Walter I. Trattner. Copyright © 1974, 1979, 1984, 1989 by The Free Press. Copyright © 1994, 1998 by Walter I. Trattner.)

Professional associations are important, for they help to raise standards and to determine the relationship between a profession and the society it serves. No, organizations of healthcare professionals are not "stuck up!" If anything, they are "stuck together," bound by a common desire to be the finest possible representatives of their profession. Within the nursing arena, there are a great number of valuable associations providing continuing education, standards and support.

Often an employer will pay your membership dues, seeing that your involvement with the professional society is to their advantage. Correspondence classes are offered by professional groups, making education affordable and easily accessible.

Among the most popular professional groups serving nursing assistants are NAGNA, The National Network of Career Nursing Assistants, National CNA Friendship Society, The Journal of Nurse Assistants and FANA.

Long-term care nurses have NADONA, ANA, American Holistic Nurses' Association, and the National Gerontological Nursing Association.

Do some research. Ask around. Find out who on staff is a member of what. Could they show you their association's newsletter? Promise yourself that, in the New Year, you will spread your wings and get involved with your profession.

TODAY: *Join an association.*

When my husband Thurmond practiced medicine, he "caught" 3,000 babies. He has always refused to say he delivered anyone, believing the mother did the work. After years of listening to expectant patients, Thurmond learned what he should expect during births. Newer, less experienced doctors at the hospital relied heavily on mechanical monitoring equipment to keep them informed during labor, but Dr. Knight always preferred his own observations and understanding.

The world is filled with knowledge and knowledgeable people. Understanding, on the other hand, can only be gained through personal experience, through applying knowledge to everyday life. Knowledge is theoretical; understanding is practical. Working in health care, we can forget the importance of consulting our own understanding of a situation.

Sure, knowing vital signs and weight loss and amount of food consumed at each meal is important, but what do you understand about your patient? Do you realize he was a night watchman, so unexpected visitors after dark get him all wound up? Or that Miss McClay is not used to having a man toilet her?

Understanding our coworkers is also important to the health and well-being of a facility. Before you judge Rowena's greasy hair, did you hear her house has been without water for two weeks?

Retreat leaders Kathleen V. Hurley and Theodore E. Dobson explain:

> Understanding comes as we recognize the truth of our negativity, self-serving motivations, and petty jealousies. Only then can we recognize and understand the same struggles in others. Awareness of self creates compassion, forgiveness and healing, gifts we first give to our self and create a new sense of identity. Then we become compassion, forgiveness and healing for others.

> The weakness that we do not embrace in ourselves, we despise and attempt to destroy in another. Individual

conscious understanding is the only neutralizing force for violence and hatred.

Jesus tried to wake people up to these same realities. "Do you still not understand, still not realize?" he asked his disciples. "Are your minds closed? Have you eyes and do not see, ears and do not hear?" (Mark 8:17-18.) Notice that he doesn't ask if they have knowledge but instead inquires about understanding.

TODAY: *Understand.*

I used to joke that we were lucky to have gravity. Without it, I surely would be knocked out by one of the countless orbiting jackets my son lost growing up.

So far this winter, our house has swallowed my husband's reading glasses, the top to the ice cream maker and my new fountain pen. With just two of us at home, these disappearances are particularly annoying. I can't imagine what it is like in facilities with 100 or 200 or more residents, plus nearly the same number of staff.

In the past year I have witnessed some clever, affordable measures nursing homes have taken to reduce the loss of personal property. Simply writing initials in marker on combs, toothbrushes, basins and bedpans can reduce the chances they will sprout feet and walk away.

At Countryside Place in Mishawaka, Indiana, social service director Karen Smith-Taljaard took the whole process up several notches. Her goal was not just to reduce the losses of patient prosthetic devices, but also to eliminate such problems at her facility.

Working with a multidisciplinary group, Karen created a tracking protocol and timetable, which is put into motion the moment dentures, eyeglasses, hearing aides and the like come up missing.

Breaking the search into discreet segments with specific individuals responsible for each step, the procedure is working beautifully. A thoughtful woman with a sharp mind, Karen reports that virtually all personal prosthetics have been recovered since the protocol was implemented.

Tackling one of the perennial nursing home demons is a brave and laudable endeavor. Unable to accept the status quo, Karen decided to take it on. Eliminating the anxiety patients face when their property turns up missing is a huge contribution to their well-being. Reducing staff time and expense related to replacing lost items is a significant achievement as well.

TODAY: *Tackle a demon.*

We knew a woman who went to medical school in her forties, with two teenagers still at home. Today, Bunny is a practicing physician. Dr. Philip Gates, an orthopedist in Vermont, was an architect when he decided he wanted to be a doctor.

Choosing to advance oneself in a new direction is an exciting prospect. But too many of us only see it as too daunting, too difficult, too much work. Instead, we brood and come to resent others who achieve our dreams. Full of excuses, we hate ourselves and our circumstances.

With the advent of the Internet and online education, achieving one's goals is easier. CNAs who want to become LPNs or RNs can earn much of the credit by cyber-correspondence.

Classes are also available for advanced certification and degrees in social services, activities and management programs. All that the student needs is willpower. Those who aspire to a job which requires additional schooling wisely keep certain realities at the front of their minds:

1. I'm going to be alive anyway, so why not invest my time, not just use it.

2. If I just stopped watching television shows about hospitals and accidents I would have enough time to study for a medical career.

3. I am not pursuing this dream for myself alone. The world needs another good professional in the field.

My friend Angel Masi has been pursing a career in Chinese medicine for close to ten years. Part of her study is to study and teach rigorous martial arts. Hearing of her disciplined workout schedule, I said to her, "I wish I felt like exercising all the time like you do. My problem is, I just don't feel like it a lot."

"Bethany," she said, looking directly at me, "I don't feel like it a lot either. I do it because I have a goal."

Deciding to climb an academic mountain is a demanding course, but clearly worth the effort. Advising those who need hope against the odds, His Holiness the Dalai Lama said:

Firstly, believe in the truth...the main thing is to work hard for that, because it is really worthwhile. It is important to get a feeling that my life is something meaningful. Then make efforts on the basis of compassion, nonviolence, and for the benefit of everyone.

TODAY: *Climb a mountain.*

I returned to the states from a peace pilgrimage in India on this date in 1998. If America is my mother, then India is my lover. I am never so happy as I am in India, and this trip was an incredibly spiritual month away from home.

After shopping for a few stocking stuffers at our country store, I ran home and announced, "Thurmond, I swear something has changed in this country while I was gone. People are so incredibly kind and genuinely friendly, it feels like I'm still in India!" With great patience, my husband explained, "Dear, it is the Christmas season, the Christmas spirit."

So Thurmond was right in that instance, but have you noticed that something is happening in this country, and December is no longer the only month for giving? For the past five years, charitable giving has risen steadily, up 40 percent. Companies are routinely giving a percentage of their profits to charity, and some employers have philanthropy committees to decide where to donate funds.

Could the nation be catching the spirit that has filled health-care facilities for years? Looking for meaning, are individuals and families seeking connections on a deeper level?

When it comes to charitable acts, caregivers are clearly the experts, leading the community in giving of self. Giving is not confined to contributing to the United Way or the Salvation Army. For caregivers, their time and their talent is part of their tithe to the community at large.

Watch the papers for the next announcement of a major corporate donation to a good cause. Send a letter signed by the staff to the generous company, welcoming them into the elite fellowship of caregivers. After all, they are following in your footsteps. Invite them to drop by and learn what you do, 365 days a year, 24 hours a day. Let them know that, if they or their family ever need quality care, you are there.

TODAY: *Praise charitable acts.*

As many churches experience a drop in attendance, outreach and mission work can also suffer. For creative activities and social service staff, these changes are challenging, nothing more. What new kinds of partnerships and programs can be developed?

For residents who receive little or no mail, pre-addressed birthday cards can be provided to a congregation, asking folks to write a little note, sign and mail on a certain date. Even the busiest of citizens usually has time for such sharing.

Sunday school classes can be invited to meet at the facility, with a promise of free refreshments served by the residents. Interested residents can sit in on the class, providing them an opportunity to enjoy the company of children.

Due to budget constraints, the church no longer has a secretary. Could your front office handle the church's Vacation Bible Day Camp registrations? In exchange, would the campers present a play for residents?

Jill Trewin, the activities director from the Detroit area who wrote the introduction to this book, encourages churches to become involved with her facility. One of the local churches has sponsored a Bus Ministry for residents. Twice a month, church members arrive in their bus to transport any and all able-bodied nursing home residents to attend the church service and enjoy a home-cooked meal. Church members have had basic training in how to assist frail elders, which reduces everyone's anxiety and increases the joy. A few volunteers even became certified as aides.

Begin a conversation with churches in your neighborhood. How can you help one another?

TODAY: *Create church partnerships.*

Bonnie Sparks, a nursing home chaplain in Sandusky, Ohio, has planned a most amazing Christmas Eve for the residents of her facility and a nearby group home for displaced youth.

With the aid of her lay ministers, other volunteers and her daughter, Pastor Bonnie has put together a Christmas Eve sleepover for the children at the nursing home. The kids will sleep in the chapel, and wake to a Christmas morning with all the trimmings, hosted by the nursing home residents.

Observing religious holidays and other traditions anchors our lives. Following death, divorce or other tragedies, children and adults can feel lost and disconnected from their past. Staying in a convent a few weeks before Christmas, I met a young woman who was recovering from a nervous breakdown. The pressures of college had proven to be too much. Now, Kristin was beginning the slow journey toward recovery. Her speech was flat, and her eyes seemed glassy and far away. The third night of her stay, Sister Rosalie told her she was needed in the kitchen.

A few hours later, Kristin came bouncing down the hall. "Look, we decorated Christmas cookies!" she sang out. Through such a simple ritual, her broken spirit was on the mend.

Your facility is full of individuals who have suffered pain, hardship and disappointment in the past year. Young mothers and fathers have lost custody or perhaps visitation with their children. Older residents know that no relative will drop by to celebrate the holidays. Yet, all want to experience the healing traditions of Christmas, to decorate cookies and string popcorn.

How can you help restore a coworker or resident to wholeness? What single holiday tradition can you share to make a spirit bright?

TODAY: *Share a tradition.*

Learning Christ:

Teach me, Lord, to be sweet and gentle in all the events of life: in disappointments, in the thoughtlessness of others, in the insincerity of those I trusted, in the unfaithfulness of those on whom I relied.

Let me put myself aside, to think of the happiness of others, to hide my little pains and heartaches, to that I may be the only one to suffer from them.

Teach me to profit by the suffering that comes across my path.

Let me so use it that it may mellow me, not harden nor embitter me; that it may make me patient, not irritable; that it may make me broad in my forgiveness, not narrow, haughty and overbearing.

May no one be less good for having come within my influence. No one less pure, less true, less kind, less noble for having been a fellow traveler in our journey toward Eternal Life.

As I go round from one distraction to another, let me whisper, from time to time, a word of love to Thee. May my life be lived in the supernatural, full of power for good and strong in its purpose of sanctity.

—From La Salette Seminary Aid Society,
Shrine of Our Lady of La Salette, Altamont, NY

TODAY: *Live for a good purpose.*

Helen was a ball of energy and one of the charter members of the Florida Association of Nurse Assistants. A conscientious aide, Helen wanted to apply for a promotion to physical therapy assistant, but didn't feel she was worthy or qualified. FANA Founder Terry Bucher recalls:

> In speaking with Helen, I noted her strengths: willingness to learn through attending our education programs, a true love for her residents and an ability to adapt to new situations. I encouraged her to fill out an application for the position and accept an interview.

Following the interview, Helen bubbled over with enthusiasm.

> Terry, do you know what made the biggest impression on the interviewer? It was the fact that, of my own initiative, I had taken the time and interest to be a better CNA, through attending monthly education programs. They couldn't believe I would do this on my own accord.

Today, Terry holds this memory of Helen dearly:

> That moment was a real joy for me as I recognized Helen's sense of pride and self-esteem. She has since died of breast cancer, and the memory of her pride after that job interview continues to serve as a source of encouragement to me in my work with nursing assistants.

Long-term care is a funny business. Virtually everything we do is mandated by the government, a condition we regularly squawk about. Everyone resents the heavy hand of regulation, dictating everything. Yet without these outside standards, how many caregivers would imitate Helen and pursue training?

Because tax dollars and lives are at stake, government is compelled to intervene. Let's get beyond complaining about the regulations, and look at our own standards and goals. Is it time to learn some more?

TODAY: *Attend education.*

"Oh, you look just like my daughter!" the frail resident called out to a stranger at the end of the hall. "For a moment, I thought you were my Susan. You look just like her."

How many of us have experienced this longing for a familiar face? In big cities, I find I am always scanning crowds, looking for a friend. My first year at the University of Michigan, which boasted 40,000 students on campus, I had never seen so many people and known so few. Never seeing anyone I knew in my daily walks across campus, I became disoriented and depressed. Not only did I not know anyone, no one knew me!

"Are you expecting your daughter?" the visitor asked Susan's mother.

"No. She lives far away. I was just hoping."

"Well, let's pretend I am Susan and have a big hug!" The grateful resident burst into tears and fell into the stranger's arms. "You know, I can't be near my mother today, either, so this is great for me, too, Mom," the stranger said to her new relation.

Studies have shown more than half of the residents of nursing facilities have no local family. Yet this statistic does not eliminate the natural craving residents have for visits and contact with family. Consider the lives of those in your care. Are there some folks who rarely, if ever, get a visit? Can you become an almost-family-member for them?

TODAY: *Be family.*

Caregivers in large healthcare institutions walk miles and miles each day. Sitting down is a rare luxury.

Perhaps the nature of your work is what makes the typical fundraisers for health organizations so ironic: the Memory Walk for Alzheimer's, the March of Dimes Walk, the Heart Association Walk, the Breast Cancer Walk. As if anyone needs to walk some more!

Hardly a weekend goes by during the summer and fall months that someone isn't walking for something, seeking a pledge to support their trek.

Strangers sometimes think caregivers are nuts, spending more time on their tired feet, parading down the city streets for yet another good cause. But watching the nursing home delegation laugh and joke, your participation isn't all that hard to understand.

The secret of most caregivers is that they don't think of work as a job-not like others do. Taking care of others is an expression of self, which also happens to be a source of employment. Caregivers go to work because they need to be themselves. Yes, they may try working somewhere else, but they always come back.

Highly aware of the ravages of most diseases, caregivers are quick to join a walk that fights AIDS or MS or CP or any other destroyer of life. Having buried too many favorite patients who were crippled and consumed by fatal illnesses, caregivers are eager to support research and cures.

The next time you walk for a cause, get the residents to make you some crazy hats or tie-dye some T-shirts. Call the media and let them know you are walking again for health and life. Kind of like what you do every other day of the week.

TODAY: *Walk.*

Dedicated caregivers speak of their career or profession. Recognizing one's standing in the world of work is an important step in valuing yourself. Far from being a temporary or casual laborer, you are a respected healthcare provider.

Is your career something that "just happened?" A fluke? Hardly! No matter how you first entered the field, the real measure of your dedication is found in the reason you stayed. Most people who begin a job as a nursing assistant leave. It's called turnover and you see it every day. Why did you stay?

Because you heard an inner call—a call not just to a career but to a vocation:

> Vocation is another term that has been used to characterize a person's lifework. It, too, has undergone considerable change as we have moved into the modern world. As early as Martin Luther's time the word-it means 'calling'-was used principally to refer to people in religious life: mostly monks and nuns. His transformation of the use of the term to the widest applications has always been deeply meaningful. Luther proposed that every person's work be considered a proper vocation. 'Why,' Martin Luther said, 'A man could cobble shoes to the greater glory of God.'

In a world of 24-hour quadraphonic sound, with Dolby speakers in every corner and car, hearing an inner call isn't always easy. The world is forever shouting its competing messages, promoting the job that pays the most, regardless of the duties.

Take this moment to appreciate your good fortune, as well as your obedience. Recognize that your own commitment to others is grounded in a sacred call to serve, as old as life itself. If mankind is to survive, it will be because people like you answered the mysterious call to value life. Thank you.

TODAY: *Celebrate your vocation.*

As we know, Florence Nightingale's journey to become a nurse was not an easy one. Prohibited from becoming a caregiver by her parents, Florence rebelled at age 32, when she headed off to Turkey with 37 other women to care for victims of the Crimean War.

Conditions in Scutari were frightful. The square-shaped hospital, a converted barracks comprised of four one-mile corridors, was devoid of furniture—not even a table for surgery. Thousands of soldiers were frostbitten, starved, wounded and dying of cholera when Florence arrived in 1855. The outhouses at the end of each corridor were overflowing, rats were everywhere, and the daily allowance of water for all purposes was one pint a head.

The doctors were given orders by the British government to admit but not employ the nurses, so Florence and her crew were prohibited from being near patients. Because the doctors had absolute power, the women set to work on sorting linen and making pillows, stump rests and slings, while suffering and dying men went unattended.

For days no invitation came from the doctors, while wounded poured into the already-full hospital. Barred from entering the wards, Florence turned her attention to the feeding arrangements. Many of the wounded and sick men were literally starving, and others were being killed trying to eat ill-cooked solids when they should have been on an invalid's diet.

On day ten, with men dying by the hundreds, the nurses were granted entry. Can you imagine the frustration? And the dedication? To have waited 15 years to become a nurse, and then to be denied access to patients? And the resistance did not end there.

"When in March 1855, a quantity of bedding and utensils arrived, Dr. McGrigro had them immediately installed in the wards. But they had not been through the proper channels and Dr. Cummings ordered them to be removed." As one of the doctors said to Florence, "It is not a question of efficiency, nor of the comfort of the patient, but of the Regulations of the Service." To keep her temper and her purpose in the face of all this inefficiency, timidity and intrigue, and when she herself was subject to such extremes of fatigue, must have required almost superhuman self-control.

Considered the Mother of Modern Nursing, Florence Nightingale's example guides us well beyond the nuts and bolts of care. More than ninety years after her death, we continue to be inspired by her persistence, vigilance and clear forward thinking.

TODAY: *Be vigilant.*

An old folk tale relates the story of the rich boy who answers his front door and finds a hungry poor boy, begging for food. "Get out of here, you bag of rags!" the rich boy screams, slamming the door. From the kitchen, his mother hears what has happened, and calls her son in.

"Show me how the good boy inside you would have answered that door," she asks.

With little hesitation, her son softens his face and says, "Come in, poor neighbor, and let us give you a meal."

"From now on, please have only the good boy inside answer our door," his mother instructs.

Hearing this story, all children immediately begin to nod; they know the good boy. How and why do human being share this common inner knowledge, this touchstone? Rabbi Harold Kushner answers:

> You will notice that when you carry out acts of kindness, when you pray, study, give to charity or forgive someone who may have hurt you, you get a wonderful feeling inside. It is as though something inside your body responds and says, 'yes, this is how I ought to feel!'

> Why do we get this wonderful feeling? I believe that each of us was put on this earth to fulfill his or her potential for humanity, and the soul is that part of us that makes us truly human. The soul is what makes a human being a human being and not simply another living creature on God's earth. The soul is not a physical entity, but instead refers to everything about us that is not physi-cal-our values, memories, identify, sense of humor. Since the soul represents the parts of the human being that are not physical, it cannot get sick, it cannot die, it cannot disappear. In short, the soul is important. When you fulfill your soul's destiny, you will feel 'right.'

(Reprinted with the permission of Little, Brown and Company, from "God's Fingerprints on the Soul" by Harold Kushner. Copyright © 1996.)

TODAY: *Fulfill your destiny.*

References

January

17 - Submitted excerpt from page 23 from *Wisdom, Distilled from the Daily; Living the Rule of St. Benedict Today* by Joan Chittister. Copyright © 1990 by Joan D. Chittister. Reprinted by permission of HarperCollins Publishers, Inc.
21 - Helen M. Luke, *Dark Wood to White Rose: Journey and Transformation in Dante's Divine Comedy*, (Parabola Books, 1993).
23 - Thomas Keating, *Open Mind, Open Heart, The Contemplative Dimension of the Gospel*, (New York, The Continuum Publishing Co., 1998), 94-99.
24 - Walter Trattner, *From Poor Law to Welfare State: A History of Social Welfare in America*, (New York, The Free Press, 1999), 217, 277.
25 - National Interfaith Committee for Worker Justice, press release, Chicago, April 9, 1999.

February

6 - Lorene Hanley Duquin, *The Life of Catherine de Hueck Doherty, They Called Her The Baroness*, (St. Paul, Alba House, 1995), 284-285.
15 - *American Journal of Psychiatry* 155 (1998): 536-542.
22 - Andre Dubus, excerpt from *A Father's Story*, from *The Times Are Never So Bad* (David R. Godine, Publisher, Inc. 1983).

March

6 - John Briggs, *Fire in the Crucible: Understanding the Process of Creative Genius*, (Phanes Press, 2000), 201.
12 - State of Vermont Department of Aging and Disabilities Commissioner David Yacovone, speech, March 1998.
15 - Submitted excerpt from page 102 from *Wisdom, Distilled from the Daily; Living the Rule of St. Benedict Today* by Joan Chittister. Copyright © 1990 by Joan D. Chittister. Reprinted by permission of HarperCollins Publishers, Inc.
16 - James F. Birren and Donna E. Deutchman, *Guiding Autobiography Groups for Older Adults: Exploring the Fabric of Life*, (Baltimore, Johns Hopkins University Press, 1991).

17 - Briggs, p. 271.

19 - Carl Gustav Jung, *Modern Man In Search of A Soul,* (New York, Harcourt Brace Jovanovich, 1933), 108.

22 - Colleen L. Johnson and Leslie A. Grant, *The Nursing Home in American Society,* (Baltimore, Johns Hopkins University Press, 1985).

23 - Submitted excerpt from page 85 from *The Crone: Woman of Age, Wisdom and Power* by Barbara G. Walker. Copyright © 1985 by Barbara G. Walker. Reprinted by permission of HarperCollins Publishers, Inc.

April

3 - Henri J.M. Nouwen, *The Road to Daybreak, A Spiritual Journey,* (New York, Doubleday, 1988), 351.

6 - Briggs, p 233.

7 - Ibid, p 256.

11 - Florence Nightingale, *Letters and Reflections,* (Evesham, UK, Arthur James Ltd., 1996), 64.

12 - Elwood N. Chapman, *Attitude: Your Most Priceless Possession,* (Menlo Park, CA, Crisp Publications, 1995, distributed by National Book Network 1-800-462-6420).

16 - Trattner, p. 33.

19 - Karen Thomas, "Children Fantasize About Riches," *USA Today,* 22 January 2001.

20 - Submitted excerpt from page 131 from *What's My Type? Use the Enneagram System of 9 Personality Types* by Kathleen V. Hurley and Theodore E. Dobson. Copyright © 1991 by Enneagram Resources, Inc. Reprinted by permission of HarperCollins Publishers, Inc.,

26 - Dr. V. Tellis-Nayak, "DONs: A Resource in Peril" (presentation at the 51st Annual Convention and Exposition of the American Health Care Association, Orlando, FL, October 11-13, 2000).

28 - U.S. Catholic Bishops Pastoral Letter, "Justice in the Workplace: Voices and Choices," *Arkansas Catholic,* (Catholic Committee of the South, December 9, 2000), 8-10.

May

2 - Bernie Glassman, *Bearing Witness: A Zen Master's Lessons in Making Peace*, (New York: Harmony Books, 1998), 71.
6 - Briggs, p. 28.
16 - Drew Leder, "A Modest Proposal, We Should Help Our Elders Age Gracefully," *U.S. Catholic*, April 1995, 35.
22 - Nouwen, p. 183.
23 - Child, *The Family Nurse or Companion of the American Frugal Housewife*, (Bedford, MA, Applewood Books, 1997), 12-13, 145, 147.

June

5 - Linda Sandmaier, (winning essay, Caregiver Recognition Week, Calgary Home Support Services, Calgary, Alberta, Canada, September 1, 2000).
6 - Rachel Naomi Reman, MD, "In Service of Life," Review, Institute for Noetic Sciences, Spring 1996.
9 - Briggs, p. 225.
14 - Sairose Kassam, "Home Support Worker, Growing Career Trend!"(winning entry, Calgary Home Support Services, Calgary, Alberta, Canada, September 2000).

July

4 - J.E. Esslemont, *An Introduction to the Bahá'í Faith: Bahá'u'lláh and the New Era*, (Wilmette, IL, Bahá'í Publishing Trust, 1980), 173-174.
7 - Johann Christoph Arnold, *Seeking Peace: Note and Conversations Along the Way*, (Farmington, PA, The Plough Publishing House, 1998), 7.
12 - Diann Neu, *WATERwheel*, 2, No. 1, (1989). Diann L. Neu is the co-director of WATER, The Women's Alliance for Theology, Ethics and Ritual, 8035 13th Street, Silver Spring, MD 20910. Phone: 301-589-2509, Fax: 301-589-3150; www.hers.com/water; dneu@hers.com.
13 - Glassman, pp. 41-43, 110.
15 - James Juhnke and Valerie Schrag, *The Original Peacemakers*, (Fellowship, Fellowship of Reconciliation, May/June 1998), 9.
19 - www.larchecanada.org

19 - Nouwen, p. 179.

24 - Masami Saionji, *The Golden Key to Happiness*, (Rockport, MA, Element Books, 1995), 47.

25 - Bede Griffiths, *Return to the Center* (Springfield, IL, Templegate Publishers, 1976), 125.

26 - Helen Fisher, *The First Sex: The Natural Talents of Women and How They are Changing the World*, (New York, Ballantine Books, 1999), 44.

27 - Juhnke, p. 9.

28 - Marian Edelman, "Caring Enough to Build a World of Peace," *Fellowship* (Fellowship of Reconciliation, January/February 2001), 4.

31 - Jay Miller, ed., *Mourning Dove, An Alishan Autobiography*, (Lincoln, NE, University of Nebraska Press, 1990), 148.

August

16 - Trattner, p. 60.

19 - John Robbins and Mortifee, *The Awakened Heart: Meditations on Finding Harmony in a Changing World,* (Tiburon, CA HJ Kramer 1997).

24 - Trattner, pp. 80-81.

25 - Dr. Timothy Conway, *Women of Power and Grace: Nine Astonishing, Inspiring Luminaries of Our Time*, (Santa Barbara, CA, The Wake Up Press, 1994), 323.

September

12 - Mary E. Rogers, *The Mentor*, II, no. 2 (February, 1892).

October

5 - L. Lissner, "Variability of Body Weight and Health Outcomes in the Framingham Population," *New England Journal of Medicine* 324 (1991): 1839-1844.

5 - P. Boyle, "Increased Efficiency of Food Utilization Following Weight Loss," *Physiological Behavior* 21 (1978): 261-264.

13 - Briggs, p. 280.

14 - Ha Kroeger, *The Basic Causes of Modern Diseases and How to Remedy Them*, (Carlsbad, CA, Hay House, Inc., 1998), 18-19.

18 - Mary Beth Markelin, "Female Freshman Doubt Tech Skills," *USA Today*, 22 January 2001.

21 - Trattner, p. 18.

22 - Dr. Kathleen DesMaisons, *Potatoes not Prozac*, (New York, Simon and Schuster, 1998), 28.

26 - John R. Lee, *What Your Doctor May Not Tell You About Menopause*, (New York, Warner Books, 1996), 307.

November

3 - Submitted excerpt from page 71 from *Wisdom, Distilled from the Daily; Living the Rule of St. Benedict Today* by Joan Chittister. Copyright © 1990 by Joan D. Chittister. Reprinted by permission of HarperCollins Publishers, Inc.

6 - Barbara Ehrenreich and Deirdre English, *Witches, Midwives and Nurses, A History of Women Healers*, (New York, The Feminist Press, 1993), 21, 32-33.

8 - Dr. John Bland, *Live Long, Die Fast*, (Minneapolis, Fairview Press, 1997), 3.

9 - Chaim Potok, *The Book of Lights*, (New York, Fawcett Crest, 1982), 383.

13 - Helen Fisher, *The First Sex: The Natural Talents of Women and How They Are Changing the World*, (New York, Ballantine Books, 1999), 49-50.

13 - Edgar N. Jackson, *Understanding Health: An Introduction to the Holistic Approach*, (Philadelphia, Trinity Press International, 1989), 91.

14 - Dr. Timothy Conway, *Women of Power and Grace: Nine Astonishing, Inspiring Luminaries of Our Time*, (Santa Barbara, The Wake Up Press, 1994), 247.

17 - Colette V. Browne, *Women Feminism and Aging*, (New York, Springer Publishing Co, 1998), 75.

19 - Jackson, p. 14.

20 - Philip St. Romain, *Kundalini Energy and Christian Spirituality, A Pathway to Growth and Healing*, (New York, Crossroad, 1995), 69.

26 - Caroline Myss, *Anatomy of the Spirit*, (New York, Three Rivers Press, 1996), 161.

December

1 - Barbara Ehrenreich and Deirdre English, *Complaints and Disorders: The Sexual Politics of Sickness*, (New York, The Feminist Press, 1973), 33.

2 - Specified excerpts from pages 88, 90, 93 from *Wisdom, Distilled from the Daily; Living the Rule of St. Benedict Today* by Joan Chittister. Copyright © 1990 by Joan D. Chittister. Reprinted by permission of HarperCollins Publishers, Inc.

4 - James Hilton, *Lost Horizon*, (New York, William Morrow and Co, 1933), 64.

8 - Briggs, p. 167.

11 - Briggs, p. 133.

15 - NAGNA Five Point Plan, www.nagna.org.

16 - John Robbins, *Reclaiming our Health: Exploring the Medical Myth and Embracing the Source of True Healing*, (Tiburon, CA, HJ Kramer, 1998) 240-241.

17 - Trattner, p. 151.

19 - Submitted excerpt from page 131 from *What's My Type? Use the Enneagram System of 9 Personality Types* by Kathleen V. Hurley and Theodore E. Dobson. Copyright © 1991 by Enneagram Resources, Inc. Reprinted by permission of HarperCollins Publishers, Inc.

21 - His Holiness the Dalai Lama "The Dalai Lama Speaks," (Tibet Press Watch, August 2000), 6.

29 - Eric Dean, *St. Benedict for the Laity*, (Collegeville, MN, Liturgical Press, 1989), 87.

30 - Elspeth Huxley, *Florence Nightingale*, (London, Weidenfeld and Nicholson, 1975), 77, 99.

31 - Harold Kushner, "God's Fingerprints on the Soul," *Handbook for the Soul*, (New York, Little, Brown and Company, 1996), 20-21.

About the Author

And he led them out as far as Bethany, and blessed them with uplifted hands; and in the act of blessing he parted from them. And they returned to Jerusalem with great joy, and spent all their time in the temple praising God.

—Luke 24:50-53

Author and motivational speaker Bethany Knight believes all life will be treasured, and peace will comfort the planet when the caregivers of the world tell their precious love stories.

She participated in International Way of Peace Pilgrimages to India and Northern Ireland, praying for world peace, in 1998 and 2000.

Bethany is a former long-term care ombudsman, state health care association director, and lobbyist. She has worked as a pastor, nursing assistant, and long-term care insurance agent, as well as a newspaper reporter and gubernatorial speechwriter.

Bethany and her husband, Dr. Thurmond Knight, a luthier, live on 160 acres in northern Vermont, which they've named Shantivanam (Peace Forest) after the ashram Bede Griffiths founded in southern India.

She is writing her fifth book, *Eve Within*, a novel.

To learn more, visit www.tenderlovingcalling.org.